Medical Law, Ethics, & Bioethics

FOR THE HEALTH PROFESSIONS

6 edition

Medical Law, Ethics, & Bioethics

FOR THE HEALTH PROFESSIONS

6 edition

Marcia (Marti) Lewis, EdD, RN, CMA-AC
Adjunct Instructor, Medical Assisting (Formerly) Dean, Mathematics, Engineering,
Sciences and Health
Olympic College
Bremerton, Washington

Carol D. Tamparo, PhD, CMA-A
(Formerly) Dean, Business and Allied Health
Lake Washington Technical College
Kirkland, Washington

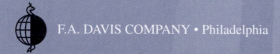

F.A. DAVIS COMPANY • Philadelphia

F. A. Davis Company
1915 Arch Street
Philadelphia, PA 19103
www.fadavis.com

Copyright © 2007 by F. A. Davis Company

Printed in the United States of America

Last digit indicates print number: 10 9 8 7 6 5 4 3 2 1

Acquisitions Editor: Andy McPhee
Developmental Editor: Jennifer A. Pine
Art and Design Manager: Carolyn O'Brien

Library of Congress Cataloging-in-Publication Data

Lewis, Marcia A.
  Medical law, ethics, and bioethics for the health professions / Marcia (Marti) Lewis,
Carol D. Tamparo. — 6th ed.
      p. cm.
  Includes index.
  ISBN-13: 978-0-8036-1730-8
  ISBN-10: 0-8036-1730-5
   1. Medical laws and legislation—United States. 2. Ambulatory medical care—Law and legislation—United States. 3. Medical ethics—United States. I. Tamparo, Carol D.,
1940- . II. Title.
  KF3821.L485 2007
  344.7304′1—dc22   2006033905

The way a book is read—which is to say, the qualities a reader brings to book—can have as much to do with its worth as anything the author puts into it.

Norman Cousins

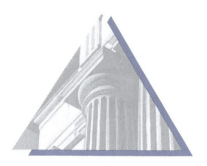

Preface

It is imperative that the health care professional have knowledge of medical law, ethics, and bioethics so that the client may be treated with understanding, sensitivity, and compassion. No matter what the professional's education and experience, any direct client contact involves ethical and legal responsibility. It also is imperative that this knowledge be used to provide the best possible service for the physician employer. Our goal is to provide the health care professional with an adequate resource for the study of medical law, ethics, and bioethics.

Although the material is applicable to all health care professionals in any setting, our emphasis continues to be on the ambulatory health care setting rather than the hospital or long-term care setting. For example, we do not address such legal and bioethical issues as whether or not to feed an anencephalic newborn in the neonatal center of the hospital because this book's focus is on the ambulatory health care setting. We realize, however, that all bioethical issues may affect ambulatory health care personnel. Continued enthusiastic feedback from instructors, students, and reviewers is gratifying and has resulted in many changes that will make this sixth edition an even more useful resource than the first five editions. We are reminded of the truth, which comes from colleagues in our respective community and technical colleges that no matter how many times a piece is written, it can always be improved.

The continuing evolution of health care, of legal and, especially, bioethical issues necessitate this revision. The material is updated throughout the book to reflect the latest developments and to reflect emerging ethical issues. The newest developments in stem cell research for treating disease and for creating new organs and tissue are included in the Genetic Engineering chapter as the legal and ethical debate 'rages.' The chapter introducing the reader to the cultural perspectives of health care continues to heighten our awareness of the importance of culture in health care. There will be additional cultural pieces when appropriate throughout other chapters as well.

The authors and their editors have made every attempt to ensure currency and pertinence of the material. However, some bioethical issues change almost daily as lawmakers and the public become actively involved and press for legislation. Even as the sixth edition goes into production, the co-authors struggle to be current as federal and state legislations clash. Further, funding issues and morality issues are being addressed in the political arena sometimes bringing to a standstill continued research and advancement in medicine. For ease of reference, pertinent codes of ethics appear in Appendix I. Appendix II offers samples of some of the legal documents clients may use in implementing decisions about health care, life, and death.

Reader response to the vignettes has been remarkable. A thought-provoking vignette appears at the beginning of each chapter. Some of the vignettes are adapted from actual case law, and for these we have provided the relevant citations. Other vignettes recount actual situations of which we are aware. The sixth edition continues to place critical thinking exercises in chapter text. For students' benefit we have included Questions for Review at the end of each chapter for increased learning. All will whet the appetite, stimulate discussion, and highlight the most pressing legal, ethical, and bioethical issues faced by ambulatory care employees.

Learning objectives designed for the educational setting precede each chapter. The Critical Thinking questions are intended to be thought provoking rather than a test of chapter contents. References are provided at the end of each chapter whereas a complete bibliography is found at the end of the text for anyone seeking additional information. Web Resources are introduced to assist the reader in further research on the Internet. "Have A Care!" has been updated and returned to the end of the book at the request of our readers. We hope that you will derive from this book a great sense of pride for your professional position in health care.

Marti Lewis
Carol D. Tamparo

Reviewers

Kay E. Biggs, CMA, BS
Coordinator
Medical Assisting Technology
Columbus State Community College
Columbus, Ohio

Carry DeAtley, MBA, CMA
Assistant Professor and Coordinator
Medical Assisting Program
Southern State Community College
Hillsboro, Ohio

John M. Ginnetti, RN, MSN, MPH
Instructor
Medical Assisting Program
Branford Hall Career Institute
Branford, Connecticut

Marilyn M. Turner, RN, CMA
Director
Medical Assisting Program
Ogeechee Technical College
Statesboro, Georgia

F. A. Davis Medical Assistant Advisory Board

Acknowledgments

It is never possible to acknowledge all persons who make contributions to the writers of a book. Completing a book requires assistance from so many individuals and sources. We wish to thank, however, a few who were especially helpful. Without them, the book would have been impossible.

F. A. Davis has a fine cadre of individuals to make a writing project pleasant. Each individual's command for excellence and thoroughness helps to create the final product. Margaret Biblis, Publisher, and Andy McPhee, Acquisitions Editor, refresh our thoughts and goals with new ideas and discerning eyes. With the assistance of Jennifer Pine, Developmental Editor; Yvonne N. Gillam, Associate Developmental Editor; Deborah Thorp, Manager of Creative Development; and Lisa Thompson, Project Editor; the thoughts, ideas, text, and presentation are all pulled together into the final book you hold in your hands. Kim Harris, Editorial Associate, monitors our budget and provides direction and support as necessary. They have been positive, encouraging, and helpful to us in all matters. Our relationship with F. A. Davis for over 28 years has always been one of high professionalism and integrity.

Students continually offer current critical thought and information on legal, ethical, and bioethical issues and act as a sounding board for all ideas. Their input and comments have influenced this product. Students continue to be our inspiration and the reason for this book!

The support of families and friends was an essential ingredient from the inception of the first edition of the book to the completion of this sixth edition. Thanks to Les and Martiann Lewis, Tom Tamparo, Jayne Bloomberg, and Duuana Warden. They relinquished their time with us so we could write. They provided encouragement when we were discouraged and celebrated with us when we were successful. Thanks, we do love you! Last, but most important: Thanks Marti! Thanks Carol!

M.A.L.
C.D.T.

Contents in Brief

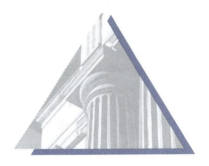

Contents

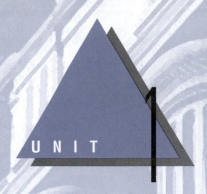

Understanding the Basics

CHAPTER 1

Medical Law, Ethics, and Bioethics

> 66 *It is much easier to find a score of men wise enough to discover the truth than to find one intrepid enough, in the face of opposition, to stand up for it.* 99
>
> *Shakespeare*

KEY TERMS

pluralistic Referring to numerous distinct ethnic, religious, and cultural groups that coexist in society.

Upon successful completion of this chapter, you will be able to:

1. Define key terms.
2. Discuss some bioethical issues in medicine.
3. Compare the terms *law, ethics,* and *bioethics.*
4. Explain the importance of ethics, law, and bioethics in the practice of medicine.
5. List and discuss at least three ethical codes.
6. Explain the Ethics Check Questions.
7. Describe the characteristics that are important for a professional health care employee.

Vignette: Are you a professional?

A certified medical assistant (CMA) employed by an obstetrician/gynecologist calls her former medical assistant instructor to inform her of an opening for a clinical assistant in the obstetrics and gynecology (OB/GYN) clinic. After describing the position and its responsibilities, the CMA says, "We really need another person in the clinical area. I'm the doctor's only nurse."

Surprised by the comment, the instructor inquires, "When did you go back to school to become a nurse?"

She replies, "Oh, I didn't, but everyone thinks I am his nurse. I do everything a nurse does."

The title *Medical Law, Ethics, and Bioethics for the Health Professions* implies three distinct topics: law, ethics, and bioethics. Such distinction however, is for the sake of clarity. These topics are integrated throughout the text. Discussing health laws without considering ethics and bioethics is nearly impossible. Conversely, discussing ethics and bioethics without considering the law is futile.

Law

Laws are societal rules or regulations that are advisable or obligatory to observe. Failure to observe the law is punishable by the government. Laws protect the welfare and safety of society, resolve conflicts in an orderly and nonviolent manner, and constantly evolve in accordance with an increasingly **pluralistic** society. Laws have governed humankind and the practice of medicine for thousands of years. Today federal and state governments have constitutional authority to create and enforce laws. A brief look at these laws, their sources, and their definitions appears in subsequent chapters.

Ethics

Ethics is a set of moral standards and a code for behavior that govern an individual's interactions with other individuals and within society. Fletcher[1] differentiates *morals* from ethics, stating, "'morality' is what people do in fact believe to be right and good, while 'ethics' is a critical reflection about morality and the rational analysis of it." According to Fletcher, for example, "Should I terminate pregnancy?" is a moral question, whereas "How should I go about deciding?" is an ethical concern.[1]

Although laws are more apt to be universal rules observed by all, different cultures have different moral codes. Therefore, there are no universal truths in ethics because it is difficult to say that customs are either correct or incorrect. Every standard for ethics is culture bound. A person's personal code has no special status; it is only one among many. See Chapter 11 for further discussion on the influence of culture.

Ethics also refers to the various codes of conduct that have been established through the years by members of the medical profession. These codes appear in the appendixes.

Bioethics

Bioethics refers to the ethical implications of biomedical technology and its practices. *Bio* refers to life, and issues in bioethics are often life-and-death issues. Ethical and bioethical standards can be personal, organizational, institutional, or worldwide.

The change in ethics related to modern medicine and research in the past few decades is most intriguing. Medicine and technology rapidly change and offer choices to clients and their families. Consumers are actively involved in their health care and more knowledgeable of medical technology and its implications. The public evaluates this technology and how it relates to their daily lives. The application of bioethics in our everyday lives provides opportunities, challenges, enthusiasm, and choices, albeit difficult, for each of us.

During former President Clinton's first term, he established an 18-member National Bioethics Advisory Commission (NBAC) with the charge to provide advice and to make recommendations to the National Science and Technology Council (NSTC) and other appropriate agencies on bioethical issues related to research. In October 2001, the NBAC charter expired. President George W. Bush, by executive order, then enacted The President's Council on Bioethics, which is under the Department of Health and Human Services. It addresses bioethical issues such as, but not limited to, ethical caregiving for the elderly, stem cell alternatives, and regulation of new biotechnologies.

Ethical Issues in Modern Medicine

Many situations arise in the practice of medicine and in medical research that present problems requiring moral decisions. A few of these can be illustrated by the following questions.

Should a parent have a right to refuse immunization for his or her child? Is basic health care a right or a privilege? Does public safety supersede an individual's right? Who dictates client care—the client, the physician, the attorney, or the medical insurance carrier? Should children with serious birth defects be kept alive? Should a woman be allowed an abortion for any reason? Should everyone receive equal treatment in medical care? Should people suffering from a genetic disease be allowed to have children? Should individuals be allowed to die without measures being taken to prolong life? Should criteria be developed to determine who receives donor organs? Should stem cell research be limited?

None of these questions has an easy answer, and one hopes never to have to deal with them. However, one may sometimes have to make these decisions or be in a position to assist those who make such decisions. These questions and possibilities are the reason for including a discussion of pertinent bioethical issues.

We do not attempt in this book to determine right or wrong for the ethical issues in modern medicine. The purpose is to present the law and the facts that are pertinent in the ambulatory health care setting and to raise some questions for consideration. Most of us have decided what *ought* to be right in each of the bioethical issues. That is important. It is also important to know how and why our opinions have been formed and to look at what is—in other words, what is acceptable according to the legal and ethical standards of today. As health professionals we must live and act so that we have respect for ourselves and for others and encourage others to have respect for themselves. We need to know what we are to become and how we can become better than we are. Even when our opinions differ from the clients we serve, clients always deserve respect and dignity from us. We hope that the forthcoming discussions on "Allocation of Scarce Medical Resources," "Genetic Engineering," "Abortion," "Life and Death," "Dying and Death" and "Have a Care" will offer a better understanding of what *is* and what may become.

In reading the following chapters and considering their effect on you personally as well as your role as a health professional, you may find the following lines from a poem by F. A. Russel (1849–1914) helpful.

REMEMBER... *Seek the right, perform the true,*
Raise the work and life anew.
Hearts around you sink with care;
You can help their load to bear.
You can bring inspiring light,
Arm their faltering will to fight.

Comparing Law, Ethics, and Bioethics

Law, ethics, and bioethics are different yet related concepts. Laws are mandatory rules to which all citizens must adhere or risk civil or criminal liability. Ethics often relate to morals and set forth universal goals that we try to meet. However, there is no temporal penalty for failing to meet the goals as there is apt to be in law. Yet most could agree that law in the United States has been the driving force in shaping our ethics.

Confusion over the definitions of law, ethics, and bioethics is understandable. Consider the following example for further clarification:

The U.S. Supreme Court addressed the issue of abortion in *Roe v Wade,* 410 U.S. 113, 1973. In law it ruled that during the first trimester, pregnant women have a constitutional right to abortions, and the state has no vested interest in regulating them at this time. During the second trimester, the state may regulate abortions and insist on reasonable standards of medical practice if an abortion is to be performed. During the third trimester, the state's interests override pregnant women's rights to abortions, and the state may deny abortion except when necessary to preserve the health or life of the mother.

The personal ethics of a physician or health care professional may dictate nonparticipation in an abortion or any abortion-related activities. Bioethics and the allocation of scarce resources are evidenced by some state statutes that have denied the use of state funds for an abortion. As demonstrated by this example, sometimes law, ethics, and bioethics conflict.

IN THE NEWS

In a continuing battle, state legislatures have rushed to tighten controls on abortions. For example, as of 2006, only Washington, Oregon, New York, Vermont, Rhode Island, Connecticut, and the District of Columbia do not have parental notification or consent laws related to minors seeking abortion. Sometimes, legislation is later overturned by the U.S. Supreme Court. Legal attempts continue to rescind *Roe v Wade*.

The Importance of Medical Law, Ethics, and Bioethics

A reasonable question is "Why are medical law, ethics, and bioethics necessary?"

 Reasons may include, but are not limited to, the following:

▲ Understand and follow health care laws.
▲ Understand the moral structure of our actions both ethically and legally.
▲ Understand and appreciate the differences in moral reasoning among individuals and groups of individuals.
▲ Understand and learn from the bioethical dilemmas that clients face.
▲ Understand our own values, morals, and ethical stances.
▲ Understand the need to confront biases and bigotry.

Factors relevant to this climate include the following:

1. Demands of society for quality health care at minimal personal cost
2. The debate over whether health care is a right or a privilege
3. The equality of the distribution and access to emerging medical technology
4. The controversy among managed care, the political arena, and the consumer about who pays for health care and how
5. The potential for greed among all participants in health care
6. The powerful role of medical insurance and managed care

Almost daily, consumers are bombarded with information on medicine and health care. The media, both printed and electronic, report on some aspects of health care. This immediate access to information causes consumers to ask more questions of the medical community and to expect to be well informed about choices. Ethical standards and laws designed to protect clients and establish guidelines for the medical profession represent efforts to create a climate for an equitable exchange between client and provider. Increasingly, ambulatory care centers are establishing ethics committees that enable community resource persons, educators, and providers to grapple with ethical dilemmas before they occur in the clinical setting. The goal of such an ethics committee is to have a plan in place before a crisis occurs.

Medical technology is advancing at a more rapid rate than either laypersons can comprehend or legal or ethical standards can address. Consider the developments in reproductive techniques. Years ago, when a woman wanted a baby, her options were readily defined. Now, with continual advancements in medical technology, her options have greatly increased. A woman desiring a child can, for example, be impregnated artificially. Such choices have their advantages and disadvantages. What influence, if any, should the doctor have in presenting these choices to the mother-to-be? Are there any problems for an offspring? Who should be involved in the decisions? Do state laws differ regarding such matters? Ambulatory health care employees need to be aware of the ethical and legal implications of such choices.

Medical specialization means more people will be involved in personal health care. Managed care, policies, and providers will in part dictate how choices are made. If hospitalization is necessary, who is in charge, who coordinates, and who approves this care? Who decides the appropriate course of action in the case of conflicting medical opinions? Although specialization may enhance quality health care, it demands greater coordination for clients to benefit from it, and it increases the cost of medical care.

In 1940, a normal delivery cost $35 for 10 days of inpatient hospital care. The delivering physician received an additional $35. In 1990, a normal delivery cost an average of $3300 for a 2- to 3-day inpatient hospital stay. In 2005, hospitalization for normal delivery and a 1- to 2-day hospital stay was $5250 (Fig. 1–1). Such figures are difficult to track because of the numerous and varied contracts in managed care. Query your classmates and friends for today's costs of a normal delivery. In 1996, Congress forced health insurance to provide a minimum of a 48-hour hospital stay for normal delivery.

According to the U.S. Census Bureau report, *Income, Poverty, and Health Insurance Coverage in the United States*, 46 million Americans have no health care coverage, an increase that is statistically significant. That constitutes 15% of the population. Medicare and Medicaid now pay less of the total bill for the elderly and the indigent than was origi-

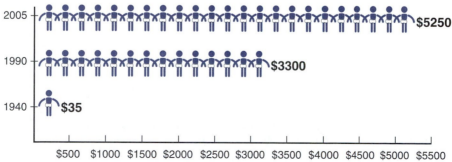

FIGURE 1–1 Comparison of hospital care for normal delivery during the last 65 years.

nally planned, and many of the working poor who hold down one or more part-time jobs do not qualify for medical benefits. At the same time, managed care is instituting every cost-saving measure possible, thus dictating to providers what and how costs will be covered.

For example, a 47-year-old man requiring surgery for a hernia reported to the hospital operating room in the morning and was discharged to his home the evening of the operation because his insurance would not cover an overnight stay. His wife, untrained in nursing care, had to take 2 days' leave from work to care for him. As the burden of quality health care costs shifts back to consumers, states struggle to pass laws regarding the equitable distribution of health care dollars and additional ethical concerns raised over that distribution.

Oregon's Basic Health Care Services Act of 1989 is an example of how a state sought to expand coverage and access to health care by extending Medicaid eligibility to most Oregonians below the federal poverty line. Further, the law identified basic health benefits for all persons in the state. The problem, of course, is the realization that in providing basic health care for all Oregon residents, choices were made that identified those procedures to be covered and those to be eliminated, both a courageous and controversial move (see Chapter 12). Oregon continues to revisit the original Basic Health Care Services Act to greater address consumers' needs. At least four other states seek to provide health care to all residents.

Codes of Ethics

Professional codes have evolved throughout history as practitioners grappled with various ethical and bioethical issues. Increasingly, groups of professionals have defined how members of their profession ought to behave.

The Hippocratic oath (see Appendix I), although not prominent in medical schools today, still may be found on the walls of many health care settings and clinics. The oath, which was first written in the fifth century B.C..., became Christianized in the tenth or eleventh century A.D. to eliminate reference to pagan gods. The Hippocratic oath protected the rights of clients and appealed to the inner and finer instincts of the physician without imposing penalties.

The Geneva Convention Code of Medical Ethics, established by the World Medical Association in 1949, is similar to the Hippocratic oath. This code refers to colleagues as brothers and states that religion, race, and other such factors are not a consideration for care of the total person. This code reflects the fact that medicine was becoming available to all during this era.

The Nuremberg Code was established between 1946 and 1949 as a result of the trials of war criminals after World War II. This code suggests guidelines for human experimentation and is directed to the world. The writers hoped that the code would ensure the safety of humans in the years to come.

IN THE NEWS

The wars in Iraq and Afghanistan caused ongoing debate about abuse of both the Geneva Convention and Nuremberg Code by military personnel on all sides of the conflict. One example is the highly publicized abuse of prisoners in the Abu Ghraib prison. How does the reported abuse of the prisoners challenge the terms of the Geneva Convention and Nuremberg Code?

The Declaration of Helsinki, written between 1964 and 1975, is an update on human experimentation. Much more detailed than the Nuremberg Code, it includes guidelines for both therapeutic and scientific clinical research. Unlike the Nuremberg Code, the Declaration of Helsinki is directed to the world of medicine rather than the world at large.

The Medical Assistant Code of Ethics (see Appendix I) is directed to the medical assistant and to office and clinic assisting. The code was adopted by the American Association of Medical Assistants and appears in its constitution and bylaws.

The American Medical Association established the Principles of Medical Ethics in 1847 and updated it in 1957, 1980, and again in 2000 (see Appendix I). The preamble and nine principles have served as guidelines for physicians for many years. The document "Current Opinions of the Judicial Council of the American Medical Association" is intended as an adjunct to the revised Principles of Medical Ethics. Both documents are pertinent to physicians and their assistants today.

Other codes have appeared that deal more with the rights of clients than the responsibilities and guidelines for health care providers. They include numerous Patient Bill of Rights established by federal and state governments as well as individual hospitals and institutions. The purpose of these documents is to inform clients of their rights. Clients have always had these rights, but might not have been aware of them.

An Ethics Check

 Blanchard and Peale,[2] in *The Power of Ethical Management,* developed a set of questions to serve as an "ethics check" that is a useful tool for persons facing an ethical dilemma. The ethics check suggests that ethics is a very personal concept and personal decision.

A personal code to adopt might include Blanchard and Peale's three questions:

1. Is it legal or in accordance with institutional or company policy?
2. Does it promote a win–win situation with as many individuals (client/employee/employer) as possible?
3. How would I feel about myself were I to read about my decision or action in the daily newspaper? How would my family feel? Can I look myself in the mirror?

If the answer to any one of the three questions is no, the action is unethical. If the answer to all three questions is yes, the action is ethical. The clarification of our own personal code of ethics helps clarify actions; however, these ethics check questions might further clarify how to act when in a difficult situation.

An individual will have great difficulties remaining ethical in an organization that is unethical. It helps if the leader of a group is ethical, making it easier for everyone else to be ethical. However, ethical actions may come from anyone, regardless of status.

▲ CRITICAL THINKING EXERCISE

You are the office manager in a large multiphysician medical center. There is no upward mobility in this center, and you relish a new challenge. It is a rather slow day, and you use your office computer to access the Internet to do a job search. You find four that are exciting, and you send your resume on the Internet. As you disconnect from the Internet, you recall that it is easy to trace access to sites on the Internet. Apply the ethics check.

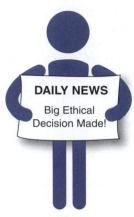

FIGURE 1–2 An ethics check: How would I feel if I saw my decision in the newspaper?

Characteristics of a Professional Health Care Employee

The significant conflict that often arises among law, ethics, and bioethics mandates that individuals choosing health professions be persons of high moral standards. They should be clear, open, and knowledgeable about their personal choices and beliefs and be able to recognize vast diversity in a pluralistic society. Health care professionals must feel comfortable in a "servant" role while maintaining their own integrity and the respect of their clients.

Individuals employed in a service-oriented industry such as health care are expected to have certain characteristics. The health professional must always be tactful and should know instinctively when speaking is wise and when listening is better. The health care employee is an important communication link between the client and the physician.

Anyone in a health care profession is in a nonreciprocal relationship with clients. The professional serves the client and gives the client full respect even when the client is disrespectful. Health care professionals will be nonjudgmental of their clients and their activities, offering information rather than opinions. Clients expect to be treated with courtesy and understanding. Only the most caring and sensitive of employees can handle day after day of sick, hurting, and complaining clients and remain objective yet compassionate.

Physician-employers require that their employees be diligent and knowledgeable in every detail of the job. Such knowledge and training can come only through professional preparation that is demanding and exacting and that is continued throughout employment. Professionals who are flexible and take initiative will be an asset to their employers.

Honesty and integrity are traits required of the employee. Physicians' employees must remember to practice only within the scope of their professional training and under the direct supervision of the doctor, never misrepresenting themselves. Refer to "Are You a Professional" at the beginning of the chapter when a Certified Medical Assistant calls herself a "nurse" when, in fact, she is not a nurse. Confidentiality must be tenaciously protected, and both the clients' and the physicians' best interests must be guarded.

Wise and prudent health care employees will select employers for whom they have respect and to whom they can remain loyal. Matching your personal understanding of "standard of care" to that of your employer avoids conflicts at a later time. The majority of health care professionals have a concern for quality health care, and that concern is often reflected in community efforts and contributions.

Persons who have these traits are successful health care employees who will find their profession rewarding and fulfilling. There is no opportunity for boredom in such a fast-paced and rapidly changing field as health care.

Summary

Knowledge of law, ethic, and bioethics is essential for all health care employees. The ethics check questions offer one approach to address these issues on a personal level. Professional codes of ethics are further guides to performance as a health care professional.

QUESTIONS FOR REVIEW

1. Define and give an example of law.

_____

_____

_____

_____

2. Define and give an example of ethics.

_____

_____

_____

_____

3. Define and give an example of bioethics.

_____

_____

_____

_____

4. Describe the scope of the President's Council on Bioethics.

_____

_____

_____

_____

5. Why do we study medical law, ethics, and bioethics.

_____

_____

_____

_____

6. List and explain the three ethics check questions.

_____

_____

_____

_____

7. Name four characteristics of a professional ambulatory health care employee.

_____

_____

_____

_____

CLASSROOM EXERCISES

1. State in your own words what ethics, law, and bioethics mean to you.

2. What is the difference between law and ethics? Can a law be unethical? Can an ethic be unlawful? Justify your response.

3. What would you do if your ethics do not agree with those of your physician-employers?

4. Do the Medical Assistant Code of Ethics and the Principles of Medical Ethics have any conflicting views? Explain.

5. In a small group discussion, tell how you as a health care professional would show respect for a client who is rude and disrespectful to you.

6. What will you do if your opinions differ from your clients? For instance, a mother refuses inoculations for her child and you believe they are necessary.

7. Using your favorite Internet search engine, key in the words "world medical ethics codes." Identify the results.

REFERENCES

1. Fletcher, J: The Ethics of Genetic Control Ending Reproductive Roulette. Prometheus Books, Buffalo, NY, 1988, pp xiii–xiv.
2. Blanchard, K, and Peale, NV: The Power of Ethical Management. Wm Morrow, New York, 1988, p 27.

WEB RESOURCES

▲ American Association of Medical Assistants (AAMA). www.aama-ntl.org
▲ American Medical Association (AMA). www.ama-assn.org

CHAPTER 2

Medical Practice Management

" *I couldn't repair your brakes, so I made your horn louder.* "

Steven Wright

KEY TERMS

bond An insurance contract by which a bonding agency guarantees payment of a specified sum to an employer in the event of a financial loss to the employer caused by the act of a specified employee; a legal obligation to pay specific sums.

burglary Breaking and entering with intent to commit a felony.

capitation Health care providers are paid a fixed monthly fee for a range of services for each HMO member in their care.

conglomerate A corporation of a number of different companies operating in a number of different fields.

co-payment A medical expense that is a member's responsibility; usually a fixed amount of $5 to $20.

deductible A cost-sharing arrangement in which the member pays a set amount toward covered services before the insurer begins to make any payments. Typically, HMO members do not pay deductibles.

fee-for-service Pays providers for each service performed.

gatekeeper A term referring to HMO primary care providers responsible for referring members to specialists with the intent of matching the client's needs and preferences with the appropriate and cost-effective use of those specialists' services.

group practice Type of business management in which three or more individuals organize to render professional service and share the same equipment and personnel.

health maintenance organization (HMO) Prepaid health care services rendered by participating physicians and providers to an enrolled group of persons.

joint venture A type of business management where hospitals, physicians, and clinics form to offer client care.

liability The state of being liable, responsible, legally bound or obligated, as to make good any loss or damage that occurs.

14

managed care A type of health care plan; generally one of two types, namely HMO or preferred provider organization (PPO).

opt-out option Members or clients can seek treatment from providers outside the health care plan but pay more to do so.

partnership Type of business management involving the association of two or more individuals who are co-owners of their business.

Pay for Performance (P4P) A type of managed care to encourage providers to improve the quality of their clients' care, and reimburses them for their progress toward a fixed goal.

preferred provider organization (PPO) A type of business agreement between a medical service provider and an insurer organization in which the fees for specific services are predetermined for an already established group of clients assigned to or selected by the provider.

professional service corporation Specific type of corporation in which licensed individuals organize to render a professional service to the public. Such licensed individuals include physicians, lawyers, and dentists.

sole proprietorship Type of business management owned by a single individual.

theft Actual taking and carrying of someone else's personal property without consent or authority and with the intent to permanently deprive a person of it.

LEARNING OBJECTIVES

Upon successful completion of this chapter, you will be able to:

1. Define key terms.
2. Compare types of medical practice management.
3. List two advantages and two disadvantages of each of the types of practice management for both the physician and the employee.
4. Compare personnel needs in each of the types of practice management.
5. Describe managed care options.
6. Discuss the role of health maintenance organizations (HMOs).
7. Discuss joint ventures and preferred provider organizations (PPOs).
8. Define the concept of general liability for physicians.
9. Identify physicians' responsibilities to employees in medical practice management.

Vignette: How did this happen?

It is 9 p.m. Thursday and you are sitting at your desk in the Midway Medical Clinic. Everyone else has gone home. Your work is not done yet; you sit back to reflect on the past 30 years. You started here as a Medical Assistant when it was a two-physician partnership. The practice grew and many changes were made. Soon there were five physicians, multiple staff and specialists, and a corporation had been formed. Because of your tenure and willingness to expand your education and responsibilities, you became the office manager. You love this job and your bosses. You are continually frustrated by the fact that you have so little time to do what you really enjoy as an office manager. Now you find yourself managing the practice and all the finances for the physicians and staff. It is more than a full-time job for you to keep track of all the insurance organizations and contracts including PPOs, federal and state reimbursement programs. As manager you want to make sure that your employers and the clinic's clients are well served.

Physicians have traditionally practiced as sole proprietorships, as partners with other physicians, as members of health maintenance organizations (HMOs), and as shareholder/employees in professional service corporations. Increasingly, however, many physicians practice in a complicated combination of more than one type of medical practice management. Which type of business management to select is an early decision made by a physician entering practice but changes throughout one's career.

Even though the business organization may change from time to time and dictate a change in certain legal questions, the physician-employer, like any other employer, incurs general **liability** for the activities of the business. General liability includes making good any loss or damage related to the business such as liability for **theft** or fire and the safety of employees and premises.

Changes in medical practice management will have an impact on health care employees and their work. Changes will be seen in the medical records, billing and accounting procedures, payroll, number and duties of employees, and benefits. Health care employees need to be aware of how the type of business organization affects them and their jobs.

Sole Proprietors

A **sole proprietorship**, or single proprietorship, is a business owned by a single individual who receives all the profits and takes all the risks (Fig. 2–1). It is the oldest form of business and is the easiest to start, operate, and dissolve. Even sole proprietors, however, are likely to function in one or more health maintenance insurance programs as preferred providers and in other types of business management. Physicians serving as sole or single proprietors of their ambulatory health care settings are becoming increasingly uncommon. There are advantages and disadvantages to this form of business management.

Advantages of Sole Proprietorships

The advantages of a sole proprietorship include simplicity of organization; being one's own boss; being the sole receiver of all profits that are generally larger than any other forms of business management; and having lower organizational costs, greater flexibility in operation, and fewer government regulations than other forms of business management.

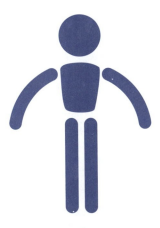

Sole Proprietor

FIGURE 2–1 Graphical representation of a sole proprietorship.

To illustrate the advantages of the sole proprietorship, consider the example of a physician who is able to establish a practice in a community by purchasing or renting facilities, to make decisions without consideration of partners or other business colleagues, and to incur minimal organizational costs. The physician also will not have to divide the profits with any other person and will be able to run the practice exactly as desired. When participating as a preferred provider in a **health maintenance organization (HMO)**, however, the physician must follow the guidelines of the HMO but does have free choice about whether to participate.

Disadvantages of Sole Proprietorships

The sole proprietorship, however, does have disadvantages. For instance, physicians may have difficulties raising sufficient capital to begin or expand the business. Medical equipment is among the most expensive of any type of equipment in a new business. The profits of the business may be insufficient to allow for expansion. In addition, physicians must know that if the business fails in a sole proprietorship or if a liability claim surpasses their insurance protection, their personal property may be attached, and they may lose virtually all personal savings and possessions. The sole proprietor typically performs all or most of the managerial functions in the business and works more than a standard 40-hour workweek.

Consider again a physician who has sufficient capital when entering practice to establish the office as a sole proprietorship. Initially, the system works well while the client load is light. However, the physician soon finds that time is at a premium when working 70 to 80 hours a week carrying a full client load and managing the business aspects of the practice as well.

Considerations for the Health Care Employee

The sole proprietor will probably begin with just one assistant. This person will need training in all areas of administrative and clinical tasks to be performed in the health care setting and will afford variety in his or her work. Although some assistants enjoy the opportunity to use all their skills in the whole operation, others may find this situation less attractive and prefer that the physician allow certain tasks to be sent outside the office for completion. These tasks might include laboratory work, transcription, correspondence, or billing and coding. The sole proprietorship often uses the services of an accountant for quarterly and yearly tax reports.

The sole proprietorship offers little if any opportunity for advancement for its employees. Therefore, the physician has to reward employees with pay raises and benefits to encourage them to remain as employees or bear the expense of hiring and retraining new employees. Physicians will select employees carefully on the basis of their education, training, and experience; reward them sufficiently for their work; and encourage them to stay a long time with the practice. Many office assistants may prefer the sole proprietorship because of the opportunity they have to make decisions and assume leadership responsibilities.

▲ CRITICAL THINKING EXERCISE

The 64-year-old sole proprietor, family practitioner, is the only physician in a rural community with a population of 3500. The physician works 70 hours a week and many weekends. He wants very much to retire or to lessen his load. What can he do?

Partnerships

A **partnership** is an association of two or more persons who are co-owners of a business for profit (Fig. 2–2). Partnerships may have only two or three members, but there is no limit to the number of individuals who may enter into a partnership. The organization may take many forms and should be defined in a partnership agreement.

The agreement should be written and reviewed by an attorney. It should include such items as the kind of business to be conducted or services to be performed, the kind of partnership being established, authority held by each partner, length of the partnership agreement, and capital invested by each partner. The agreement should also include a description of how profits and losses are to be shared, how each partner is to be compensated, limitations on monetary withdrawals by a partner, accounting procedures to be followed, procedures for admitting new partners, dissolution of the partnership, and, of course, the signatures of the partners involved in the agreement.

Some advantages of partnerships are easily recognized. Generally, a partnership has more financial strength than a sole proprietorship. Partners are likely to bring additional managerial skill and a sharing of the workload. The organization of a partnership remains relatively simple, although somewhat more complicated than a sole proprietorship.

When a physician is deciding how to establish a practice, the partnership may be desirable. If the practice is already established, only a small capital investment may be required in the beginning. This investment can be increased as the physician becomes more financially secure. A sole proprietor often will turn to a partnership when the workload of the practice requires a second person to share the work.

A disadvantage of a partnership is that two or more people make the decisions, depending on the partnership contractual agreement. A partner may not be the only "boss." In addition, each partner is responsible for the business. If one partner lacks the personal finances to assume a full share of any loss, the other partners are required to make good the deficit. If the partnership fails, usually one partner can be liable for all of the partnership debts, regardless of the size of the investment.

Personality differences should be considered because compatibility is important in any partnership. A trial period that allows a partner to withdraw from the association or be asked to withdraw after a given period may be advantageous.

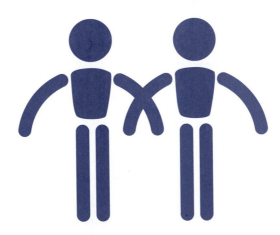

Partnership

FIGURE 2–2 Graphical representation of a partnership.

If the doctor does not wish to enter a partnership agreement but needs additional help, another physician may be hired strictly on a salary basis. Although this arrangement does not constitute a partnership, a contract may be desirable for the protection of each party.

A partnership should consider hiring more than one assistant in the health care setting because of the increased workload. Each partner may desire an assistant, but many tasks will be common to each and are best performed by one person. Assistants must understand the partnership relationship and the line of authority. Open communication on the part of all members of the staff is essential. Otherwise, each physician may expect an assistant to function as a member of the staff but may not provide input as to how this should be done.

In addition, with more than one employee, both job advancement and job specialization are possible. For example, the newly formed partnership hiring a second assistant may want to name the first assistant office manager with a specific set of duties or to assign one assistant to administrative tasks while the other performs clinical duties.

Professional Service Corporations

A corporation is a legal entity that is granted many of the same rights enjoyed by individuals. These include the right to own, mortgage, and dispose of property, the right to manage its own affairs, and the right to sue and be sued (Fig. 2–3). Physicians in a **professional service corporation** remain personally liable for their acts of medical malpractice, however, physicians are not liable for the professional acts of their colleagues. Corporations are costly to establish, more formal than either the proprietorship or partnership, and require a legal document for formation and operation.

Professional service associations or professional corporations are designed for professional persons such as physicians, lawyers, dentists, and accountants. These corporations can be identified by the letters SC (service corporation), PC (professional corporation), PSC (professional service corporation), Inc. (incorporated), and PA (professional association), depending on state law. The professional service corporation is the most intricate of all forms of medical practice and can be formed by one or more individuals.

Advantages of Professional Service Corporations

Advantages of professional service corporations include the fact that contributions to pension or profit-sharing plans can be made for all employees, including the physician. Such funds are deducted by the corporation from its taxable income, are invested, and accumulate in tax-free trusts until a future time of disbursement. Taxes are not paid on the funds until the time of their disbursement, usually at retirement, when the individual is in a lower tax bracket.

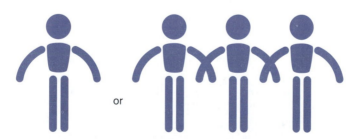

Professional Service Corporations

FIGURE 2–3 Graphical representation of a professional service corporation.

Another advantage is the corporate medical reimbursement plan. Medical and dental expenses are deductible to the corporation and nontaxable to the employee. This can result in substantial savings to both corporation and employee. Group term life insurance on a deductible premium basis is another advantage of a professional corporation. The professional corporation also may pay the professional liability premiums for physicians and their employees. Furthermore, in a corporation, physicians' personal assets are protected and cannot be attached to satisfy a debt as they can be in a sole proprietorship or partnership.

Disadvantages of Professional Service Corporations

When professional service corporations first became legal, many physicians eagerly incorporated, only to discover the disadvantages. The complexity of the professional service corporation and its detailed requirements call for reliable, well-informed attorneys and accountants to advise the corporation. The professional service corporation may be more expensive to operate than other forms of organization.

Regular meetings and agreement on organization, investments, pensions, and profit-sharing plans are important and legally required. Because more individuals generally are involved than in a sole proprietorship or most partnerships, decision-making is more complicated. Physicians often have problems finding the time to perform the functions required to run a corporation.

Although a professional service corporation usually involves two or more physicians functioning in a group setting, a sole proprietor can incorporate as a professional service corporation. The income of a single individual who incorporates needs to be sufficient to allow full participation in the benefits granted to the professional service corporation or such an arrangement is financially ineffectual.

Considerations for the Health Care Employee

The professional service corporation generally employs more assistants than a partnership or sole proprietorship. The possibility of having medical expenses covered by the corporation is an attractive inducement to prospective employees. This form of practice usually provides ample opportunity for advancement and specialization. One person should be responsible for all personnel matters to enable a smooth-running organization.

Group Practices

Another option of medical practice available to physicians is joining a **group practice** (Fig. 2–4). The physician in group practice will either be a partner, an officer of the corporation, or an employee of the practice. Most group practices are corporations, but as the workload increases, new physicians often are hired as employees.

Group practice in medicine is defined as a group of medical providers who formally organize and agree to provide medical care, consultation, diagnosis, and treatment to clients. Equipment and personnel are used jointly. The income from the group is distributed according to a predetermined agreement of the members.

  The three main types of group practice are as follows:

1. Single specialty, providing services in only one field of practice or major specialty; for example, a group of pediatricians joining together in practice
2. Multispecialty, providing services in two or more fields of practice or major specialties; for example, a group of obstetricians/gynecologists and pediatricians joining together in practice
3. Primary care group, providing services by obstetricians/gynecologists, pediatricians, family practitioners, and internists

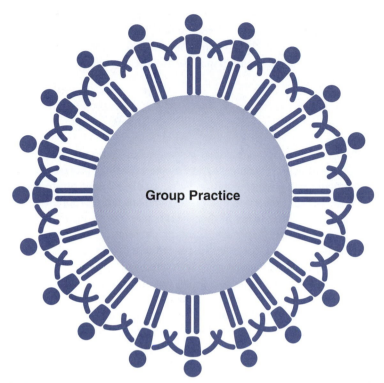

FIGURE 2–4 Graphical representation of a group practice.

Group medical practices operate on some form of **fee-for-service** basis, through insurance coverage, HMO or preferred provider arrangements, or even private pay with the same type of business arrangement as a sole proprietorship, a partnership, or a professional service corporation.

Advantages of Group Practice

Advantages to physicians in group practice include a shared financial investment for diagnostic and therapeutic equipment, the opportunity for consultation with other providers, little administrative responsibility for the practice (a group may actually employ a medical manager for the business side of the operation), and more family and recreation time because physicians in the group cover for one another. In addition, group practice may offer the intellectual and social stimulation desired by some physicians.

Disadvantages of Group Practices

The disadvantages of group practices are easily identified. Not every physician has the personality to function well in a group setting. A physician cannot act totally independent of the group and may feel a loss of freedom in such a situation. Although the working hours may not be as long as in solo practice, the income also may not be as high. Working in a close relationship with colleagues on a daily basis may lead to personality clashes and differences of opinion.

Considerations for the Health Care Employee

A group practice will have more employees than the other forms of medical organizations simply because of the larger staff of physicians and providers. Physicians generally will have less responsibility for hiring and selecting personnel, which may be an advantage or a disadvantage, depending on the physician's personal preferences. An employee may choose employment in a group for many of the same reasons as those in the corporation. Depending on the number of employees, a larger group may be less personalized.

Managed Care

Managed care is any arrangement for health care in which an organization, such as an insurance company, an HMO (see page 24), or another type of doctor-hospital network, acts as an intermediary between the person seeking care and the physician (see Fig. 2–5). Although it is not a form of business management, managed care has dramatically restructured the delivery and financial aspects of health care. No physician can practice without feeling the effects of this system. In managed care, clients, too, have experienced a radical change in the delivery of their health care. Some question the managed care corporation's financial interest in managed care. Practical information is needed to address ethical concerns that arise in the context of managed care. To fully understand managed care, a brief history of insurance coverage is warranted.

In the early 1900s, consumers expected to pay for all health care from their own pockets. During the Depression, many health care providers received little or no pay for their services. Blue Cross first provided insurance for hospital costs in the early 1930s. Blue Shield was introduced soon afterward to cover office and physician costs. Both were driven by union activity in the automobile industry.

Soon employees expected that a part of their employment benefit package would include health insurance to cover all but a few incidental and minor expenses. Increased specialization, advancing technology, and little or no emphasis on preventive care drove health care

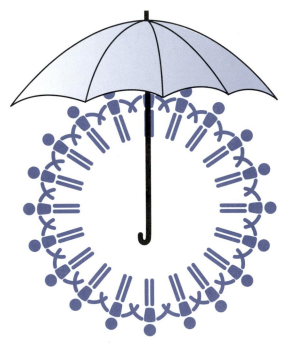

Managed Care

FIGURE 2–5 Graphical representation of managed care. Note that the umbrella covers and protects the individuals involved.

costs to a new all-time high. Employers began to struggle with the increased costs of offering health insurance to an all-demanding workforce. Health maintenance organizations (see p. 24–25) were introduced to emphasize preventive health care, assure physicians they would receive payment for their services, and ultimately begin to contain costs. It was not long before nearly every health insurance carrier was offering some form of an HMO to employees as one of the available plans.

Not all physicians and health care consumers were excited about HMOs, however. In some cases, consumers lost the right to choose their primary care physicians. The choice had to be made from a list of participating physicians. A complaint of physicians was the loss of control in the physician–client relationship. While the Health Security Bill to provide basic health care to all persons was being hotly debated in Congress and across the country, HMOs continued to grow in popularity by paying close attention to preventive care, standardizing many medical practices, and eliminating unnecessary tests and procedures. The Health Security Bill was rejected by Congress in 1994, but managed care marched on.

The method of payment for professional services changed. Instead of only the fee-for-service method of payment, in which a provider is paid for each service rendered, the **co-payment**, **deductible**, and **capitation** methods became popular.

The deductible requires policyholders to pay a set amount toward covered services on a fee-for-service basis before the insurer begins to pay claims. Providers, however, often receive only a percentage of the cost of their services once the insurer's responsibility begins.

Co-payments, a specific dollar amount paid by the client or member (usually $5–$20), were established. The co-payment helped clients realize their responsibility toward payment, but is not an amount considered too exorbitant. The co-payment adds a cash flow to the provider receiving deductible amounts and the percentage paid by insurers for remaining services.

Another method of payment, much less popular with providers, and little known and understood by clients, is capitation. Capitation gives health care providers a fixed monthly fee for a range of services for each HMO member under their care rather than a fee for each service performed. The capitation models that are most successful are placing an emphasis on the quality of care and client-satisfaction targets. In some areas, capitation plans are increasing, in other areas, they are decreasing in popularity.

A rather new form of managed care is **Pay for Performance** (P4P). P4P is a plan to encourage physicians to improve the quality of their clients' care, and reimburses physicians for their progress toward a fixed goal. Payment is dependent upon how well physicians adhere to practice standards, especially in the arenas of preventive care and management of chronic illness. P4P programs vary in their approach. Some programs pay their physicians from income received directly from participating employers or purchasers. Other programs, sponsored by managed care companies, reimburse physicians who make their target. The reimbursement rate can be as much as 5% of revenues from sponsors or purchasers. Medicare, Blue Cross, and Blue Shield are major players in P4P.

One can readily see the complexity of the problem faced by both providers and consumers in understanding the payment process and the cost of health care. What were seemingly subtle changes in the managed care contracts have had a great impact on providers and clients. Many found themselves in a form of managed care in which profit rather than health was the motive. Increasingly, providers must contact a third party for permission to perform certain procedures or make a referral to a specialist. Likewise, a client's health care services are covered when obtained from a preferred provider chosen by the insurance carrier but only partially covered or not covered at all if obtained from an unaffiliated provider. Further, some managed care plans allow members to seek treatment outside the network but charge the members more to do so. This is called an **opt-out option.**

   The problems of a business-first, client care-second system are found not only in man-aged care insurance. Covered fee-for-service plans have similar problems. The increased power of insurance carriers, which no longer simply collect premiums from subscribers and process claims, continues to take decision-making away from physicians and clients. Politi-cal influences at the state and national levels cannot be ignored either. The U.S. Congress still struggles after years of political infighting over Patients' Bill of Rights legislation that would return some control, choice, and power to clients and their physicians.

▲ CRITICAL THINKING EXERCISE

There are nearly as many varieties of managed care contracts and organizations as there is Heinz 57 sauce. It has been said that the P4P is about like putting new deck chairs on the Titanic. Explain what these statements mean to you as a health care professional, a client, or a primary care provider?

Health Maintenance Organizations

The health maintenance organization (HMO) is a dominating form of medical practice man-agement in today's society (Fig. 2–6). Kaiser Foundation Health Plan, with more than 8 mil-lion members, is the largest, not-for-profit HMO in the country. In this form of management, groups contract with clients to provide comprehensive health care and preventive medicine for prepaid fees that entitle the subscriber to service during the duration of the contract.

   The staff-model HMO owns and operates health care centers, staffed by providers con-tractually employed directly by the plan. These health care centers provide a broad range of services "under one roof," although perhaps in many locations.

   Another form of HMO allows physicians to maintain their private practices, charge their fee-for-service clients, and be reimbursed for the prepayment clients by a central HMO or-ganization. The physicians involved in this form of HMO may have clients who have prepaid for their services to any number of HMO organizations that will, in turn, pay the physician. The HMO may make use of the concept of a primary care provider (often referred to as a

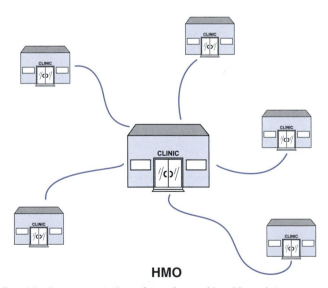

HMO

FIGURE 2–6 Graphical representation of one form of health maintenance organization (HMO). Note how the satellites extend from the main provider.

gatekeeper) as a method of controlling costs. In a gatekeeper situation, all medical care sought by a client must be channeled through the primary care provider.

The advantage to physicians who practice in a staff-model HMO is that the working hours will be regular and allow the physician more personal time. Also, such a physician will not have to provide the building or equipment necessary for practice.

Generally speaking, client and physician satisfaction with managed care services is based on personal experience. Some clients feel more satisfied; others feel less satisfied. Physicians, forced to pay more attention to the management of their practice, are generally frustrated by this additional organizational burden.

Some form of managed care or managed competition seems destined to play a role in the health care delivery system for some time to come. It should be noted, however, that in early 2000, many health care facilities and providers cancelled all their HMO contracts. This action was taken because physicians felt that the control of medical care was in the hands of managed care, not in the hands of the physician and client. Good and bad HMOs and managed care plans are no different from good and bad health care providers. Change will most likely come from informed clients who will benefit most from their health care providers. Information available through the Internet, television, public service programs, and print media will empower clients by giving them the information and vocabulary necessary to make themselves true partners in the physician–client relationship. Hopefully, a federally mandated Patients' Bill of Rights will one day provide options.

Other Business Arrangements

Today's ambulatory health care setting as a form of business management for medical practice is rapidly changing. In cities and their surrounding areas, fewer physicians are sole proprietors. However, the physician as sole proprietor may still be found in the more rural areas of the country. Larger clinics, professional service corporations, and **conglomerates** are increasingly popular.

Joint Ventures

Competition, marketing, and escalating costs have encouraged hospitals and physicians to enter into **joint ventures** that may be profitable and advantageous to both entities. For example, hospitals are building ambulatory health care settings within their service area to entice physicians to rent office space and in turn refer their clients to the hospital (Fig. 2–7). Hospitals may purchase a practice and staff it with one or more of their physicians. Such ventures provide physicians with improved marketing capabilities and fewer start-up costs.

An unusual twist to the joint venture is the establishment of in-store medical clinics in chain store markets, large and small, across the country. These chains seek such ventures to

---

IN THE NEWS

The U.S. Supreme Court unanimously ruled in *Aetna Health Inc., et al. v Davila* that the federal Employee Retirement Security Act (ERISA) precludes patients from suing HMOs in state court for injuries caused by managed care decisions. Previously, Texas legislature's 1997 Health Care Liability Act allowed patients to sue HMOs. Davila's attorney says he expects Texas patients and their attorneys to use the federal courts to challenge health plan decisions and to seek injunctions blocking health plans from denying coverage for needed treatments. Unfortunately, patients' damages will be much less because ERISA limits damages to the cost of treatment that was denied.

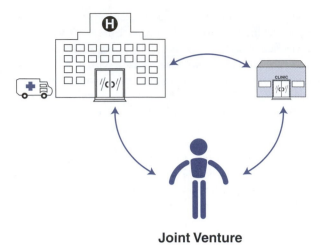

Joint Venture

FIGURE 2-7 Graphical representation of a joint venture. Note how all parties are interrelated.

increase their customer base. The in-store clinics are providing limited medical care at decreased costs and added convenience to customers.

Physician–hospital organizations (PHOs) combine hospital and group medical practices in order to offer clients a "one-stop shopping approach." A primary reason for forming a PHO is the concept that combined services are more attractive than individual services would be. In addition, both physicians and hospitals benefit one another. Clients receive more services, sometimes at a lower cost. This concept is becoming increasingly popular.

The multiple service organization (MSO) can be owned by physicians, hospitals, a totally separate party, or any combination of the three (Fig. 2–8). This organization is developed to perform physician office management services. For example, the MSO often provides secretarial and office services, billing and collections, group purchasing, and computer servicing. An MSO allows physicians to focus on client care and permits the management service to run the business side of the organization.

▲ CRITICAL THINKING EXERCISE

In a joint venture arrangement, the hospital manages three satellite clinics. In one of the clinics, there is concern that a physician assistant (PA) is spending too much time with clients. The PA is asked to log time in and time out for clients seen during a 3-week period. The PA's profitability is in question. What do you think?

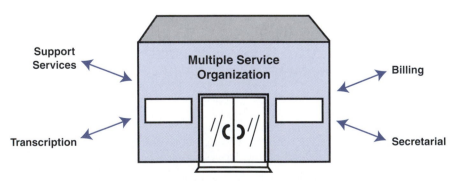

FIGURE 2-8 Graphical representation of a multiple service organization.

Preferred Provider Organizations

A provider may be a sole proprietor, a partner, or a member of a professional service corporation, as well as a preferred provider for an organization. A **preferred provider organization (PPO)** creates a contractual agreement between an insurer organization and the provider to provide medical care to an already established number of clients. For example, a physician may contract with Blue Cross's preferred provider plan to give medical care to a certain number of individuals who have subscribed to the Blue Cross preferred provider plan.

A Word of Caution

Physicians considering a move into any of the integrated organizations should be certain that the business arrangement does not violate antitrust laws. Antitrust laws exist to preserve free-market competition. Consequently, under antitrust laws any activities that restrict competition are seen as unfavorable. Physicians must ensure that the business arrangement does not oppose Medicare's fee-for-service reimbursement rules or violate any Medicare or Medicaid fraud and abuse laws. For example, because Medicare seeks a direct relationship with its providers, it may not recognize some business organizations as being eligible for Medicare reimbursement. Medicare and Medicaid laws further prohibit kickbacks and some referrals. For example, physicians cannot refer Medicare or Medicaid clients to any entity in which they have any financial interest.

More and more physicians are entering into a variety of business management arrangements, however, physicians must seek the appropriate legal advice to ensure that they are within the legal bounds of medical practice.

▲ CRITICAL THINKING EXERCISE

The large medical conglomerate provides services to health care providers in rural areas that would otherwise not have access to medical specialists. For example, a physician in a rural area can send her electrocardiograph over the phone lines and have it read by a cardiac specialist, resulting in state-of-the-art, immediate diagnosis and treatment. Can you think of another example in which medical care in rural areas can benefit from new technologies?

General Liability

Physicians engaged in business must be aware of their general liability, which includes liability for building, automobile, theft, fire, and employees' safety.

Office employees will be involved in payments of insurance premiums and submission of claims or in the establishment of physicians in practice. An understanding of the physician's general liability will be a helpful asset to any employee.

Business License

Some communities require a business or occupational license before allowing an office to be opened for the practice of medicine. Providers should check with county and city clerks to determine whether a license is required and what procedures are to be followed. An annual renewal fee may be necessary.

Building

The physician or the organization that owns the building is responsible for the building and grounds where business is conducted. If a person is injured on those premises, providers may be held legally responsible. Therefore, physicians and managing organizations carry liability insurance for the premises.

Automobile

Aside from personal car insurance, physicians may want to consider nonowner liability insurance. Such a plan protects the physician-employer if an employee has an automobile accident while performing some duty related to the business. For physicians who commonly ask their employees to make a bank deposit on their drive home or to deliver the monthly statements to the post office, such protection is wise. Whose car an employee drives makes no difference.

Fire, Theft, and Burglary

Physicians should have protection against fire, theft, and **burglary** on the building, as well as on equipment and furniture. Two types of fire insurance are most common. A coinsurance plan dictates that the owner is responsible for payment of a certain percentage of the loss, such as 20 or 30 percent. A second plan covers not only the loss but also the replacement costs. The latter is, of course, more expensive, but more beneficial in the case of loss.

Cost of protection from burglary and theft depends on location and the amount of money or valuables kept on the premises. Large amounts of money should not be kept in the office, even though most burglary attempts are made for the purpose of taking narcotics. A discussion with insurance agents will identify proper protection.

Some physicians may also insure their accounts receivable, which would be nearly impossible to recover in case of fire or loss. These items belong in a fireproof cabinet or safe after working hours to prevent their loss, even if insured.

Employee Safety

Physicians are expected to provide a safe place of employment for their employees. Safety requirements vary from state to state. Some of the variables include the number of employees, the type of employment, and the safety record of the business. Check with the state agency administering such safety regulations and workers' compensation statutes and with the state medical association to determine responsibility in this area. Refer to Chapter 10 for a discussion of regulations to protect employee safety.

Bonding

Physicians may wish to **bond** employees who are handling financial records and money in the ambulatory health care setting. Bonding is an insurance contract with a bonding agency. The purchase of a bond for a certain amount in an employee's name ensures that physicians will recover the amount of the loss, up to the amount of the bond, in case the employee embezzles funds. This precaution may be especially important when physicians do not have the time to spot-check financial transactions made by employees. Careful employers ask prospective employees if they are bondable.

Employers' Responsibilities to Employees

Whatever the style of operation in which physicians choose to practice, employers have certain business responsibilities. These include federal, state, and local requirements for Social Security compensation protection and workers' compensation for all employees. Benefits can include a uniform allowance, paid parking, medical benefits, retirement benefits, profit-sharing plans, vacations, sick leave, paid holidays and personal leave time, professional improvement allowances, and professional liability insurance.

As stated previously in this chapter, physicians must realize the value of appropriately qualified and educated employees and encourage employees to remain with the organization

---

IN THE NEWS

Is the medical practice of today too complex?

A blog posted an editorial by Jimmy K from Toronto, Ontario, June 18, 2005.

He stated, "Remember the Democrats saying how wonderful the Canadian Health Care System is and that we in the U.S. should use it as a model for our own system, (socialized medicine). Well, it seems that the Canadians have other thoughts about their system." He said that Ipsos-Reid fielded a survey of 1000 Canadian residents and found that 70% agree that they should be able to buy services from a private health care provider because they think it will lead to shorter waiting lists and improvements in the quality and availability of the health care services.

---

as long as possible. Specific information about physicians' responsibilities to employees can be obtained from an accountant or attorney. County, state, or national medical associations have information about requirements for setting up a practice and also have guidelines for employees. The AMA provides an administration pack of texts that address matters of finance, patient relations, teamwork, and day-to-day operations.

Summary

Physicians can open new practices, function as sole proprietors, be employed by other physicians on a straight salary basis, establish partnerships, become part of professional service corporations, and practice alone or in groups. Most also will be related to some form of HMO and participate in more than one form of managed health care. All forms of medical practice have advantages and disadvantages. The choice depends on the individual personality and preference of the physician. None should be entered into without advice and consideration from persons knowledgeable in the field.

The overriding factor for physicians to consider is what type of business organization will best permit them to serve their clients. Physicians must remember that the type of practice chosen will dictate their responsibilities in all areas of general liability. To be less than meticulous in this area of business potentially mars a physician's reputation.

QUESTIONS FOR REVIEW

1. The definition of a sole proprietor is
   Its advantages are

_____

_____

   Its disadvantages are

_____

_____

2. The definition of a partnership is
Its advantages are

_____

_____

Its disadvantages are

_____

_____

3. The definition of a professional service corporation is
Its advantages are

_____

_____

Its disadvantages are

_____

_____

4. The definition of group practice is
Its advantages are

_____

_____

Its disadvantages are

_____

_____

5. The definition of managed care is

_____

_____

Problems with managed care include

_____

_____

6. The definition of an HMO is
Its advantages are

_____

_____

Its disadvantages are

_____

_____

7. Define joint venture

_____

_____

8. Five types of general liability for a physician's business include:

_____

_____

CLASSROOM EXERCISES

1. What kind of business management exists in the ambulatory health care setting where you are employed or where you would be most interested in seeking employment? Justify your response.

2. Give reasons why physicians may choose a particular style of business management at different stages of their careers.

3. You are offered a position in an HMO but enjoy your present position in a sole proprietorship. What must you consider in making a decision to leave or stay?

4. You are concerned about how medical costs can be contained. Address your concern in the various types of business management.

5. What would the functions of the bookkeeper entail in an ambulatory health care setting in which the physician was a preferred provider for many separate insurers?

6. Why would a physician in an ambulatory health care setting or clinic have the bookkeeper bonded?

7. Discuss areas of concern that the issue of managed care raises.

8. In "How Did This Happen?" what options does the office manager have? What advantages does either the partnership or corporation offer her? Personally, what gains has she made as the practice grew and what has she lost?

REFERENCES

1. Bayley, C: Perspective: Pay for Performance: The Next Best Thing. Hastings Center Report, Vol. 36, No. 1, January-February 2006 (inside back cover).

WEB RESOURCES

▲ Agency for Healthcare Research and Quality. www.ahrq.gov/news
▲ American Medical Association. www.ama-assn.org
▲ Benefit News. www.benefitnews.com
▲ Healthcare Information and Management Systems Society. www.himss.org

CHAPTER

3

Employees in Ambulatory Care

" *The idea behind the tiny flower is that it really doesn't matter how small you are, whether in size or numbers. It doesn't matter how much you know, or how skilled you are. It doesn't matter how much education or how much credentials you have. What really matters is how you affect the world around you.* "

Serge Kahilii King

KEY TERMS

certification Documentation, usually from a professional organization, that an individual has met certain requirements set forth by that organization.

endorsement An agreement in which one state recognizes the licensing procedure of another state, considers it valid, and grants a license to practice. Sometimes referred to as *reciprocity*.

licensed practical nurse (LPN) or licensed vocational nurse (LVN) Person who has graduated from a 1-year practical nurse vocational or college program and has passed the state licensing examination for practical or vocational nurses. An LPN or LVN works under the direct supervision of a registered nurse (RN) or a physician.

licensure Legal permission, granted by state statutes, to perform specific acts; for instance, a physician is licensed to practice medicine.

medical assistant (MA) Person who assists the physician in both administrative and clinical duties; education varies from on-the-job training to 2 years in an accredited program for medical assisting. May be certified (CMA) or registered (RMA) by successfully passing the professional organization examination.

medical laboratory technician (MLT) Person who has graduated from a certificate program or associate degree program and then works under the supervision of a physician or medical technologist in a laboratory. May be certified by a professional organization examination.

medical technologist (MT) Person who has graduated from a 2- to 4-year college or university program in medical technology that includes 1 year of clinical training in the laboratory.

medical transcriptionist Person who may, or may not, have formal training; will have superior keyboarding and grammar skills; transcribes medical dictation, on- or off-site.

nurse practitioner (NP) Nurse practitioner is an RN (usually with a bachelor's degree) who has successfully completed additional training in an NP program at the masters or doctoral level.

physician assistant (PA) Person with 1 to 4 years of education in an approved program for PAs; a PA works under supervision of a physician.

professional coder Coders are responsible for the correct application of procedures, supplies, and diagnostic codes used for billing professional medical services.

reciprocity An agreement by which two states recognize the licensing procedures of each other, consider them valid, and grant licenses to practice based on the other state's licensure. In some states, it is referred to as *endorsement*.

registered nurse (RN) Person who has graduated from a 2-year associate degree, 3-year diploma, or a 4- to 5-year bachelor's degree program and passed the state licensing examination for RNs. An RN works under the direction of a physician.

registration An entry in an official record listing names of persons satisfying certain requirements and level of education.

LEARNING OBJECTIVES

Upon successful completion of this chapter, you will be able to:

1. Define the key terms.
2. List and define the three categories of nurses found in health care settings and compare their education and training.
3. Discuss licensure, certification, and registration of health care professionals.
4. Provide at least three examples of nonlicensed personnel in the health care setting.
5. List two similarities and dissimilarities between (1) a technician and a technologist, and (2) a physician assistant and a medical assistant.

Vignette: What would you say?

A patient is referred to a consultant for diagnosis. The consultant's receptionist secretary obtains the patient information, including the referring physician's name. The receptionist secretary is not familiar with this doctor's name, looks it up in the telephone directory, and cannot locate any information on the doctor. She comments to the patient, "I cannot find your doctor's name in the directory. He must not be licensed to practice." When the patient is examined by the consultant, the consultant makes some derogatory comments about the referring physician.

The patient later tells his primary physician what the receptionist secretary and the consultant said.

KAPLAN V GOODFRIED, 497 SW2D 101 (1973).

The number and types of employees in the health care setting vary with the practice. Generally, the more specialized the practice, the more specialized the personnel. Rarely is any health care treatment given without the involvement of a "team" of employees responsible for certain aspects of a client's care.

Employees in the health care setting may fall into the following categories: (1) those who are licensed, (2) those who are registered, and (3) those who are certified. Some employees may be none of the three, and some more than one.

Licensure is the strongest form of regulation. It requires passing a licensing examination and paying a licensing fee. A license establishes that the employee has met minimum standards required by law. Licensure laws protect the public from unqualified practitioners, and limit and control admission to different health care occupations. Licensed employees must obtain their licenses from a state authority before employment. Licensure of physicians is discussed in Chapter 5.

Registration is a process by which individuals in a particular health field are listed in a registry. This list is then available to health care providers. The state has little or no power over the registration process. There are two methods of registration. One occurs when individuals list their names in an official registry of a health area in which they work. There is no power to deny employment to unlisted persons, however, if they have sufficient knowledge and training. The second form of registration requires a predetermined level of education. Professional associations interested in recognizing qualified health care professionals administer examinations that must be passed before the appropriate credential can be conferred. This formal registry is most likely seen in ambulatory care. Registration requires payment of a fee.

Certification probably is the most common form of regulation. It occurs when a professional organization warrants that the certified person has attained a certain level of knowledge and skill, generally through a national examination. This certification of health care professionals usually exceeds the standards required of any governmental agencies. Certification is a self-regulating, credentialing process that is fully voluntary. However, this does not prevent anyone without certification from practicing. A certification fee is required (Fig. 3–1).

Licensed, certified, and registered persons may use appropriate symbols after their names to verify their credentials. Examples include the RN (Registered Nurse), CMA (Certified Medical Assistant), and MT (ASCP) for Medical Technologist (American Society of Clinical Pathologists). Both certification and registration are voluntary. Licensure is mandatory.

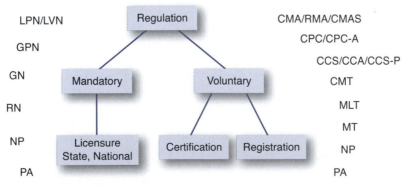

FIGURE 3–1 Not all professions follow the same regulations.

There is at least one health care profession, the **physician assistant** (PA) that may be licensed, certified, or registered. The credential of the PA will depend on the state where the PA practices and the state's statutes regarding the physician and PA. People who are not licensed, registered, or certified are also employed in ambulatory health care settings. These employees are not regulated by a professional organization. They may be trained on the job, or they may have professional training and education but choose not to attain certification or registration. For some employees there may be no certification or registration possible.

Licensed Personnel

Nurses

One of the largest groups of licensed health care professionals is nurses. Training and education for nurses fall into three categories: **licensed practical nurse** (LPN) or **licensed vocational nurse** (LVN), **registered nurse** (RN), and **nurse practitioner** (NP).

Licensed Practical Nurse/Licensed Vocational Nurse
Graduate practical nurses (GPNs) take a state board examination to be licensed as an LPN or LVN. The GPN has completed a 1-year education course at a community agency; a public vocational/technical school; or a junior, community, or senior college. The substance of this program includes nursing practices and introductory educational courses. This nurse is considered a technician. LPNs or LVNs care for the disabled, the sick, and the convalescent under the supervision of physicians or registered nurses. Most LPNs/LVNs provide basic bedside care in hospitals, nursing homes, and long-term-care facilities. They may also work in the ambulatory health care setting.

Registered Nurse
The registered nurse (RN) is the largest health care occupation, with more than 2 million jobs. Graduate nurses (GNs) from one of three types of educational programs must take the National Council Licensure Examination (NCLEX) to be licensed as an RN:

1. The diploma nurse is generally a graduate of an accredited hospital-based program lasting 2 or 3 years during which nurses engage in client care and classroom work. Direct client care and bedside experience are stressed. There are only a small number of diploma nurse programs available.
2. The associate degree nurse is a graduate of an accredited junior, community, or technical college program that awards graduates an associate degree in nursing. The college provides the educational base and condenses the practical instruction into a 2-year program. However, educational prerequisites generally take an additional year or more.
3. The bachelor's degree nurse is a graduate of a 4- or 5-year program that stresses the importance of general nursing education rather than hospital-based experience. Most administrative positions are held by bachelor's degree nurses, as are the positions of public health and school nurse.

The GN sits for the same nursing examination regardless of educational preparation identified previously. The GPN also sits for a nursing examination; however, the examination differs from that for GNs. The education and training received in all of these programs emphasize hospital or nursing facility employment.

The nurse must pass the appropriate national examination in order to use the LPN, LVN, or RN title. This license is renewed as mandated by state law. Most states require a renewal fee; some states require continuing education units (CEUs) for license renewal. Continuing education includes approved seminars, workshops, college courses, independent studies, and approved on-the-job training. Nurses must keep a record of all successfully completed continuing education classes and submit proof of completion to the appropriate agency when renewing their licenses. All nurses should know their state's requirements and recommendations. Employers should have a procedure for checking nurses' licenses annually.

Nurses wishing to practice in another state must seek **reciprocity** or **endorsement** in that state. Reciprocity or endorsement occurs when one state recognizes the licensing procedure of another, considers it valid, and grants a license to practice based on the other's licensure. If there is no reciprocity process, the nurse must satisfy the state's licensure requirement.

Nurses may be employed in offices or clinics because of their technical expertise in clinical areas. Few nurses, however, have skills relating to the business aspect of the ambulatory health care setting or have the desire to function in that capacity.

Nurse Practitioner

The nurse practitioner is an RN (usually with a bachelor's degree) who has successfully completed additional training in a nurse practitioner program at the masters or doctoral level. The NP then seeks national certification, which requires written or oral examination.

Nurse practitioners usually function independently in expanded nursing roles according to each state's nurse practice act. They may specialize and be certified in such areas as pediatrics, geriatrics, midwifery, or emergency room medicine. Nurse practitioners may examine, diagnose, and treat clients—acts formerly performed solely by physicians. This diagnosis and treatment capability often puts the nurse practitioner in the center of controversy with physicians.

The employment field for nurse practitioners varies. For instance, they may be found in isolated areas of the country managing a clinic and providing total client care, or they may be found in public health in charge of family planning clinics. Nurse practitioners also may be found in a pediatrician's office responsible for the initial history, examination, and screening of clients who are then seen by the physician.

Nonlicensed Personnel

Generally, most ambulatory health care employees are not required to be licensed or certified. These individuals include the **medical assistant** (MA), **professional coder**, **medical transcriptionist, medical technologist** (MT), and **medical laboratory technician** (MLT). Education and training vary widely among nonlicensed personnel. Many are certified or registered. All function under the supervision of the physician.

Medical Assistant

The medical assistant's (MA) versatility provides for efficient management of the entire health care setting. Although the MA is a generalist, the role may be highly specific, depending on the duties assigned.

The American Association of Medical Assistants (AAMA) defines medical assisting as "an allied health profession whose practitioners function as members of the health care delivery team and perform administrative and clinical procedures."[1] Educational and training programs for the MA are usually 1 or 2 years in a private or postsecondary vocational/technical, community, junior, or senior college awarding a certificate, diploma, or associate degree. Programs include academic courses and clinical experience. Typically, the MA receives training and education in both administrative and clinical practices.

Medical assistants may achieve credentialing through two sources. The American Association of Medical Assistants (AAMA) offers the CMA certification; the American Medical Technologists Association (AMT) offers the RMA and CMAS certification. Each requires

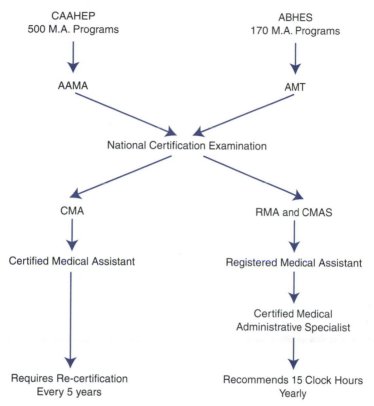

MEDICAL ASSISTANT PROGRAMS
in
PRIVATE AND POSTSECONDARY SCHOOLS

Recognized by the U.S. Department of Education

CAAHEP
500 M.A. Programs

ABHES
170 M.A. Programs

AAMA

AMT

National Certification Examination

CMA

RMA and CMAS

Certified Medical Assistant

Registered Medical Assistant

Certified Medical
Administrative Specialist

Requires Re-certification
Every 5 years

Recommends 15 Clock Hours
Yearly

FIGURE 3–2 Education and credentialing of medical assistants.

successful completion of a national examination that covers all aspects of medical assisting. The Certified Medical Assistant may then use the initials "CMA" after his or her name, and the Registered Medical Assistant may use the initials "RMA" after his or her name. Certified Medical Administrative Specialist may use the initials "CMAS" after his or her name. (Refer to Fig. 3–2.)

Accreditation of Medical Assistant Programs
The Commission on Accreditation of Allied Health Programs (CAAHEP) awards or denies accreditation to medical assistant programs (in addition to many other allied health programs). The AAMA, working in conjunction with the American Medical Association (AMA), defines the essential components and standards of quality that educational institutions must follow in educating medical assistants. Only graduates of CAAHEP-accredited medical assistant programs are eligible to sit for the national certification examination. The AAMA believes that this safeguards the quality of care to the consumer, ensures the CMA's role in a rapidly evolving health care delivery system, and continues to promote the identity and stature of the profession. Further, CAAHEP is recognized by the U.S. Department of Education.

The Accrediting Bureau of Health Education Schools (ABHES) also awards and denies accreditation to medical assistant programs in private and postsecondary institutions. The health care programs are Medical Assistant, Medical Laboratory Technician, and Surgical Technician. The American Medical Technologists, in cooperation with ABHES, define the curriculum for the programs that prepare students for the medical assisting profession. ABHES has been in operation more than 35 years, and also is recognized by the U.S. Department of Education.

The training and education of medical assistants specifically prepares them for employment in the ambulatory health care setting. However, the fact that medical assistants function as multiskilled health care practitioners places them in a strategic position for employment. Other places of employment include hospitals, medical laboratories, insurance carriers, and educational institutions. The economic and political climate in the health care arena provides opportunities for medical assistants to meet the increasing demands in any number of areas of the health care delivery system.

▲ CRITICAL THINKING EXERCISE

A medical assistant (MA) and registered nurse (RN) work side by side in a large medical setting. A recent downsizing has required assignments to be shifted. The RN is angered by the MA's appointment to an expansion of duties. There is a significant pay difference between the two salaries with the nurse's salary being higher. Discuss.

Other Employees

Physician Assistant

Physician assistants (PAs) perform functions delegated to them by physicians. In some states, PAs practice under the license of doctors of medicine or doctors of osteopathy who employ them. In other states, PAs have specific legal status such as licensure, certification or registration that details their specific scope of practice. The PA exercises autonomy in medical decision-making and provides diagnosis and therapeutic services. A physician has complete responsibility for the care of the client while the PA shares that responsibility with the delegating physician.

The educational requirements for the PA vary, running approximately 26 months. Among tasks performed by PAs are interviewing clients, taking histories, doing routine physical examinations and laboratory tasks, treating burns, suturing and caring for cuts and wounds, changing dressings, making rounds in the hospital, and prescribing and administering medications as delegated by the physician. Physicians may delegate functions only within their own competence. Physician assistants may be found in many areas. Most work with physicians in private or partnership practices in primary care, but some also work in a variety of hospital settings and in group practices.

Additional Health Care Employees

Other employees in the health care setting may include the medical receptionist, medical secretary, medical transcriptionist, book-keeper, insurance biller and coder, medical laboratory technologists/technicians, and phlebotomists. The tasks performed by these individuals are no less important than the others mentioned. Their training and education vary from on-the-job training to formal education. Four disciplines are specifically identified here: the certified medical transcriptionist (CMT), professional coders, medical technologist (MT), and medical laboratory technician (MLT).

The CMT is a transcriptionist who has passed the national certifying examination given by the American Association of Medical Transcriptionists. A CMT may be employed in the ambulatory health care setting, but a large clinic is more likely to hire a full-time transcriptionist. A smaller facility may employ a transcriptionist part time or on a contract basis as the need arises. Increasingly, medical transcriptionists are employed in multiservice organizations, and they may work at great distances from their employer.

An emerging and important health care profession is the professional coder. Coders are responsible for the correct application of procedures, supplies, and diagnostic codes used for billing professional medical services. Without accurate medical documentation and the correct coding, reimbursement will be lessened or even denied. There are approximately 44,000 professional coders in the country. There are two associations that credential professional coders. They are as follows:

▲ American Academy of Professional Coders (AAPC) that includes certified professional coder apprentice (CPC-A), certified professional coder—hospital apprentice (CPC-HA), certified professional coder (CPC), and certified professional coder—hospital (CPC-H).
▲ American Health Information Management Association (AHIMA) that includes certified coding associate (CCA), certified coding specialist (CCS), certified coding specialist—physician based (CCS-P).

Medical technologists and medical laboratory technicians are nonlicensed personnel who may be found in the ambulatory health care setting. The difference is that MTs require little to no supervision and often supervise technicians. MTs can perform complex analyses, fine-line discrimination, and error correction. MTs receive 4 to 5 years of college education including clinical training. MLTs receive their education through either a certificate or associate degree program varying in length from 1 to 2 years. They conduct and perform tests on tissues, cells, and fluids, then summarize data and send it to the physicians or providers for their review.

Considerations for Ambulatory Care Employees

REMEMBER... All employees of ambulatory health care need to continue their education. Obviously, continuing education benefits not just the individual and the employer but also, and more importantly, the welfare of the clients they serve. Many health care professions require continuing education to maintain their licensure, certification, or registration. Employers should have a procedure for making certain all employees are up to date in their credentialing.

State regulations vary and will continue to change as medicine becomes more specialized. In some states, MAs cannot perform venipuncture. Some states also regulate who can practice radiography and who can administer medications. All states regulate laboratory procedures and protocol. A physician-employer must understand regulations pertinent to those individuals in his or her employ. Employees also have the professional responsibility to understand regulations pertaining to their jobs. Practicing within the law is essential for the protection of all concerned. Employers must recognize that hiring employees with appropriate qualifications and credentials helps ensure that clients receive the optimal level of quality care.

IN THE NEWS

The Medical Board of California in their October 2002 Action Report responded to physicians' interests about who may perform what type of cosmetic procedures. In response to who may use lasers or intense pulse light devices to remove hair, spider veins, and tattoos, they state:

"Physicians may use lasers or intense pulse light devices. In addition, physician assistants and registered nurses (not licensed vocational nurses) may perform these treatments under a physician's supervision. Unlicensed medical assistants, licensed vocational nurses, cosmetologists, electrologists, or estheticians may not legally perform these treatments under any circumstances, nor may registered nurses or physician assistants perform them independently, without supervision."

In response to who may inject Botox, they state: "Physicians may inject Botox, or they may direct licensed registered nurses, licensed vocational nurses, or physician assistants to perform the injection under their supervision. No unlicensed persons, such as medical assistants, may inject Botox."

Watch for action in other states regarding these issues.

Summary

When considering the education and training of various health care professionals, one must remember that each is a vital link in the chain to quality health care. No one functions independently of any other. Each health professional has skills and responsibilities to complement every other health professional. When competition and territoriality cause conflict between professionals, quality health care is diminished. The education, training, and scope of practice for each health care professional are specifically and purposely designed to complement rather than to conflict.

QUESTIONS FOR REVIEW

1. The following are the three types of nurses and their education:

_____

_____

2. The definition of a physician assistant is

_____

_____

3. The definition of a medical assistant is

_____

_____

4. Compare and contrast the education, training, and certification for CMA, RMA, and CMAS.

_____

_____

5. Explain the difference between the MT and MLT.

_____

_____

6. Describe a CMT.

_____

_____

7. Define the responsibilities of a professional coder.

_____

_____

CLASSROOM EXERCISES

1. *Case A:* A solo family practitioner is setting up a practice in a small, rural community. *Case B:* Six physicians are entering a group practice in a city of 40,000. Specialties include obstetrics/gynecology, family practice, internal medicine, and pediatrics. What number and kinds of employees would you recommend in case A? In case B? Explain your choices.

2. What kind of medical practice is most likely to employ a
   a. PA
   b. MA
   c. Nurse practitioner?

3. Discuss the similarities and differences among licensure, certification, and registration.

4. Consider the AAMA definition of a medical assistant. Change that definition to include any state regulations peculiar to your area.

5. Increasingly, large health facilities are asking health care professionals to do more with less. Some are approached about becoming a specialist in a particular area with or without additional training or education. For example, a CMA may be asked to become an emergency room (ER) technician with specialized, in-house training. Or the same person may be asked to be a surgical technician with the appropriate training and education. Others may be asked to work in an entirely different role outside their education and training. What are the legal and ethical implications of such requests? Discuss.

REFERENCES

1. American Association of Medical Assistants: "The Scope of Practice of the Medical Assisting Profession. www.aama-ntl.org/ed

WEB RESOURCES

▲ American Academy of Professional Coders. http://ww.aapc.com
▲ American Health Information Management Association. http://ahima.org
▲ American Medical Technology Association. www.amtl.com

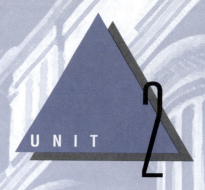

Law, Liability, and Duties

CHAPTER 4

Legal Guidelines for Health Professionals

"The virtue of a man ought to be measured, not by his extraordinary exertions, but by his everyday conduct."

Pascal

KEY TERMS

administer a drug To introduce a drug into the body of a client.

appellant One who appeals a court decision to a higher court.

arraignment The procedure of calling someone before a court to answer a charge.

civil case Court action between private parties, corporations, government bodies, or other organizations. Compensation is usually monetary. Recovery of private rights is sought.

closing arguments Summary and last statements made by opposing attorneys at a hearing or trial.

Controlled Substances Act Federal law regulating the administration, dispensing, and prescription of particular substances that are categorized in five schedules.

court of appeals Court that reviews decisions made by a lower court; may reverse, remand, modify, or affirm lower court decision.

court order An order issued only by a judge to appear or to request certain records. The release of any records requested in a court order does not require the client's permission.

criminal case Court action brought by the state against individual(s) or groups of people accused of committing a crime; punishment usually imprisonment or a fine; recovery of rights of society.

cross-examination Examination of a witness by an opposing attorney at a hearing or trial.

defendant The person or group accused in a court action.

deposition A written record of oral testimony made before a public officer for use in a lawsuit.

direct examination Examination of a witness by the attorney calling the witness at a hearing or trial.

dispense a drug To deliver controlled substances in a bottle, box, or some other container to the client. Under the Controlled Substances Act, the definition also includes the administering of controlled substances.

examination of witness Questioning of a witness by attorneys during a court action.

expert witness (medical) Person trained in medicine who can testify in a court of law as to what the professional standard of care is in the same or similar communities.

felony A serious crime such as murder, larceny, assault, or rape. The punishment is usually severe.

higher (superior) court The court to which appeals of trial court decisions can be made; a court with broader judicial authority than a lower or inferior court.

judge A public official who directs court proceedings, instructs the jury on the law governing the case, and pronounces sentence.

jury Six to 12 individuals, usually randomly selected, who are administered an oath and serve in court proceedings to reach a fair verdict on the basis of the evidence presented.

law Rule or regulation that is advisable or obligatory to observe.

litigation A lawsuit; a contest in court.

lower (inferior) court Usually, the court in which a case is first presented to the trial court; a court with limited judicial authority.

misdemeanor Type of crime less serious than a felony.

opening statements Statements made by opposing attorneys at the beginning of a court action to outline what they hope to establish in the trial.

plaintiff The person or group initiating the action in litigation.

prescribe a drug To issue a drug order for a client.

probate (estate) court State court that handles wills and settles estates.

sentencing Imposition of punishment in a criminal proceeding.

small claims court Special court intended to simplify and expedite the handling of small claims or debts.

subpoena An order to appear in court under penalty for failure to do so.

subpoena duces tecum A court order requiring a witness to appear and bring certain records or tangible items to a trial or deposition.

summons An order, in a civil case, from the court directing the sheriff or other appropriate official to notify the defendant where and when to appear.

verdict Findings or decision of a jury.

LEARNING OBJECTIVES

Upon successful completion of this chapter, you will be able to:

1. Define key terms.
2. Explain in a brief paragraph why knowledge of the law is necessary for health professionals.
3. Describe the source of law.
4. List the three branches of government in the United States.

5. Give an example of each of the following terms: (a) *constitutional law,* (b) *common law,* (c) *statutory law,* (d) *administrative law,* (e) *plaintiff,* (f) *defendant,* (g) *felony,* and (h) *misdemeanor.*
6. List two similarities and two dissimilarities between criminal and civil law.
7. Review, in diagram form, the process for (a) a civil case, (b) a misdemeanor case, and (c) a felony case.
8. List the three steps necessary for obtaining a narcotics registration.
9. Describe in outline form the office procedure to follow for administering and dispensing controlled substances.
10. Recall the five schedules of controlled substances and give an example of each.
11. Diagram the federal court system and state court system.
12. List two factors that determine in which court a case is heard.
13. Discuss the use of probate and small claims courts.
14. List two similarities and two dissimilarities among a subpoena, *subpoena duces tecum,* and court order.
15. Explain, in your own words, the trial process.
16. Name two circumstances that might require the services of an expert witness.

Vignette: Can she be an expert witness?

As a medical assistant educator with several years of experience in the administrative area and a recognized authority on medical records, you have been asked to testify as an expert witness regarding protocol for making corrections in a medical record. You agree.

When you are interviewed by the attorney and given the records to review, you recognize that the person responsible for the data entered in the record is a former student and a practicing certified medical assistant. It appears obvious that the records have been altered after the fact.

The U.S. legal system is complex and multifaceted. It can baffle even the most astute citizen. Physicians and members of their staff may be served subpoenas, calling them to court as defendants. They may also be called to serve as expert witnesses. Basically, there is one federal legal system and 50 different and unique state legal systems, all created by federal and state constitutions. Most legal actions pertinent to health care occur within the state and local systems.

Sources of Law

Law encompasses rules derived from several sources. The Constitution of the United States provides the highest judicial authority. Adopted in 1787, it provides the framework for our government. The Constitution, federal law, and treaties take precedence over the constitutional law of the states. The Constitution of the United States is a legal document that defines the structure and function of federal, state, and local government.

 The federal government has three branches: (1) the legislative branch is the lawmaking body, that is, Congress; (2) the executive branch is the administrator of the law and includes the president; and (3) the judicial branch is the judges and courts, including the Supreme Court. Each branch provides a system of checks and balances for the other two. For example, the power of lawmaking belongs to Congress, but the president can veto its legislation and the judiciary is empowered to review legislation. Congress, in turn, can investigate the president and control the appellate jurisdiction of the federal courts. No one branch has absolute authority. In addition to the federal government, each state has a constitution defining its own specific governing bodies. All powers not conferred specifically on the federal government are retained by the state, yet states vary widely in their assumption of that power.

Types of Law

The two basic types of law are common law and statutory law. *Common law* was developed by judges in England and France over many centuries. It emerged from customs, the ways things were done over time in England and in France. Common law was brought to the United States with the early settlers. Common law, views decided by judges, is always evolving as established principles are tested and adapted in new case situations, and also is called *judge-made law* or *case law*.

Many of the legal doctrines applied by the courts in the United States are products of the common law developed in England (or in the case of Louisiana, from France). This is a body of law based on judicial decisions that attempts to apply general principles to specific situations that arise. Common law has the force of statutory law, although it is not enacted by the legislature.

Congressional and state legislative bodies enact rules (laws) known as legislative or *statutory law*. These laws make up the bulk of our laws as they exist today. Publications containing these statutes are known as *codes*. Statutory laws may not conflict with federal law. An example of a statute pertaining to health care is a medical practice act, which defines and outlines the practice of medicine in a given state.

Legislative bodies, however, do not have the time or knowledge to enact all laws necessary for the smooth functioning of the government. Thus administrative agencies are given the power to enact regulations that also have the force of law. This type of law is called *administrative law*. The Internal Revenue Service and Federal Trade Commission are examples of administrative agencies. Both implement extensive rules in their areas of concern.

Administrative law, an extension of statutory law, affects the health care employee. The state health department, the state board of medical examiners, and the state board of nurse examiners are administrative agencies that dictate rules and regulations for health care. Further, licensing and accrediting bodies, as well as federal government programs such as Medicare and Medicaid, directly influence many policies, procedures, and functions of health care and fall under the category of administrative law. The Drug Enforcement Agency, an administrative agency of the Department of Justice, enforces the **Controlled Substances Act.**

▲ CRITICAL THINKING EXERCISE

State laws cannot override federal laws, yet states may enact a statute that does just that (i.e., South Dakota's recent decision to deny most abortions, and Oregon's action to allow physician-assisted suicide). What happens when that occurs? Discuss the "checks and balances" that exist in the United States.

Civil and Criminal Law

Law may also be classified as civil, criminal, international, and military. International and military law are not considered here. This book concentrates on civil and criminal law because of their importance in the health care setting. Figure 4–1 provides a brief overview of the trial process.

Civil Law

 Civil law affects relations between individuals, corporations, government bodies, and other organizations. Restitution for a civil wrong is usually monetary in nature. The bulk of law dealt with in health care is civil in nature.

In a **civil case,** the party bringing the action **(plaintiff)** must prove the case by presenting evidence that is more convincing to the **judge** or **jury** than the opposing evidence, a preponderance of evidence. The procedure for a civil case is shown in Figure 4–2. The plaintiff's complaint is filed in the proper court, usually by an attorney for the plaintiff. The **defendant** is formally summoned, prepares an answer, and files it in the court. If the defendant fails to answer the **summons** within the prescribed time, the plaintiff will win the case by default and judgment will be entered against the defendant.

The case may be disposed of without a trial. For example, the complaint may be dismissed because of some technical error, the summons may have been improperly served, or the complaint may not have set forth a claim recognized by law. The parties also may decide to settle out of court.

▲ CRITICAL THINKING EXERCISE

Consider, for example, a "slip, trip, and fall" case. Fran enters her physician's office, slips, and falls as she approaches the reception desk. She suffers a simple fracture of the left femur. When the receptionist comes to her aid, they discover that a snag from the rug caught the heel of Fran's shoe. Fran later takes civil action and sues her physician for medical fees and loss of employment wages for the time she was unable to work as a result of her injuries. As the plaintiff, she must prove that her physician (the defendant) was negligent. How might this case be settled in a civil suit?

Criminal Law

Criminal law pertains to crimes and punishment of persons violating the law. Criminal law affects relations between individuals and government.

 Criminal wrongs are acts against the welfare and safety of the public or society as a whole. Criminal acts usually result in a punishment of imprisonment or a fine.

A **criminal case** is brought by the state against individuals or groups of people accused of committing a crime. The prosecuting, district, or state attorney prosecutes the charge against the accused person (defendant) on behalf of the state (plaintiff). The prosecution must prove that the defendant is guilty beyond a reasonable doubt. In other words, the prosecution must be able to prove to the satisfaction of the court that a criminal act was, beyond reasonable doubt, committed by the accused.

A crime is a **felony** or **misdemeanor** that is statutorily defined. Felonies are more serious crimes and include murder, larceny (thefts of large amounts of money), assault, and rape. Gross misdemeanors or misdemeanors are considered lesser offenses. These include disorderly conduct, thefts of small amounts of property, and breaking into an automobile. The misdemeanor and felony case processes are shown in Figures 4–3 and 4–4, respectively.

The Trial Process

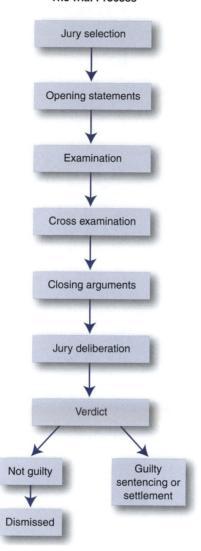

FIGURE 4–1 A general example of the trial process.

In a misdemeanor case (Fig. 4–3), the prosecuting attorney is made aware of violations of the law either by traffic or police citations, by police arrest, or by citizen information. When the prosecutor determines that enough evidence is present, the court arraigns the person on the prosecutor's charge. The charged person may plead guilty and consequently face **sentencing.** The guilty person may be put on probation, may serve a jail term or pay a fine, or may go through the appeal or appellate process. If the charged person pleads not guilty, a trial date is set. At the end of the trial, a **verdict** is given of either guilty or not guilty. If the person is found not guilty, the charge is dismissed. If found guilty, the person faces probation or a jail term or must pay a fine. The guilty person **(appellant)** may also use the appellate process.

The felony case process is shown in Figure 4–4. When evidence exists that a crime may have been committed, the police begin their investigation. Then the information is either

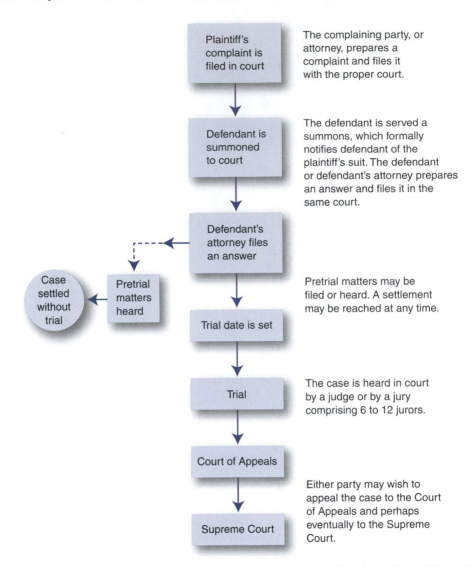

FIGURE 4–2 Chart explaining the procedure for a civil trial, which helps the public understand the judicial system in that state. Check for similar brochures in your state. (Adapted from A Citizen's Guide to Washington Courts, Washington State Office of Administrator for the Courts, 1997.)

filed by the prosecuting attorney or given to a grand jury, depending on the practice of the particular jurisdiction and severity of the charge. If the evidence is sufficient, the individual is charged. Pretrial proceedings, to plan the manner in which cases will proceed, are generally informal in nature, and many cases are settled at this point.

If the accused pleads guilty, he or she is sentenced to imprisonment, probation, or a fine. The appellate process then may be available. If the person pleads not guilty, the trial is set, the facts of the case are determined, the principles of law relating to those facts are applied, and a conclusion as to guilt or innocence is reached. If the verdict and judgment are guilty, the individual goes through the same sentencing process as in the guilty plea. If the verdict is not guilty, the person is acquitted.

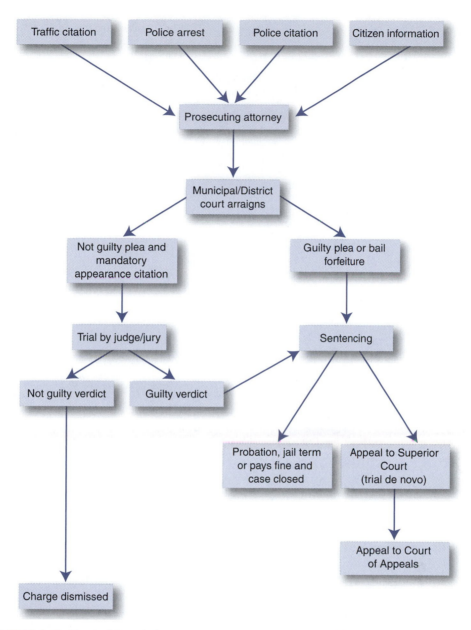

FIGURE 4–3 Chart of the misdemeanor case process. (Adapted from A Citizen's Guide to Washington Courts, Washington State Office of Administrator for the Courts, 1997.)

▲ CRITICAL THINKING EXERCISE

To illustrate both civil and criminal law, consider the following situation. Drunk driver Bill is involved in an automobile accident that causes the death of a home-maker who has two children. Bill is charged by law enforcement officials with in-voluntary manslaughter and reckless driving while speeding and intoxicated. The courts later find Bill guilty. This is criminal law protecting society. Taking this situ-ation a step further, the husband of the homemaker sues Bill for a substantial mon-

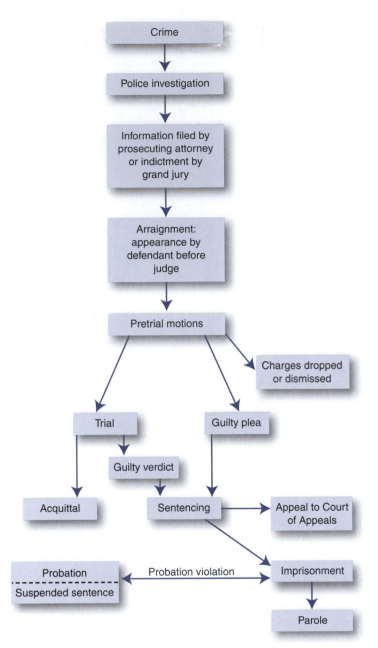

FIGURE 4–4 Chart of the felony case process. (Adapted from *A Citizen's Guide to Washington Courts*, Washington State Office of Administrator for the Courts, 1997.)

etary amount to care for the two children, who are now without a mother. On the basis of the facts of the case, the court grants a monetary award. This is civil law. Identify similar actions that you are aware of in your locale.

Controlled Substances Act and Regulations

A law all physicians strictly adhere to is the Controlled Substances Act, which regulates addicting medications. Many medications administered, prescribed, or dispensed by physicians do not fall under the Controlled Substances Act. Nevertheless, following federal guidelines for controlled substances when handling other medications is prudent, even though regulations regarding the drugs outside these schedules may be less restrictive.

The information that follows has been summarized from two main sources: Drug Enforcement Administration: Physician's Manual, ed 6. U.S. Department of Justice, Washington, DC, 1990, and Code of Federal Regulations, Title 21, Parts 1300–end, Office of the Federal Registrar, Washington, DC, 2001.

The Drug Enforcement Administration (DEA) of the Department of Justice is responsible for enforcement of the Comprehensive Drug Abuse Prevention and Control Act of 1970, more commonly known as the Controlled Substances Act.[1] These drugs are controlled because of their potential for abuse and dependence. (Substance abuse is discussed in Chapter 6.) The Controlled Substances Act lists controlled drugs in five schedules (I, II, III, IV, and V), which are discussed in detail later in this section.

The Controlled Substances Act and the *United States Code of Federal Regulations* are important to all physicians but are especially pertinent to those who will **administer a drug, prescribe a drug,** or **dispense a drug** that is listed in the five schedules. Requirements for physicians include registration, record keeping, inventory, and proper security.

Registration is with the DEA and can be completed on the Internet at www.deadiversion.usdoj.gov/index.html. Initial application is made on DEA form 224. Renewal (Form 224a) and registration changes can also be done on the Internet at the same site. A number is assigned to each legitimate handler, and registration is renewed every 3 years. Generally, a re-registration application is mailed by DEA to the registered handler approximately 60 days before the expiration date of the registration. If the application is not received within 45 days before the registration expiration, notice of such fact and request for forms must be made in writing to the Registration Unit of the DEA.

A separate DEA registration is granted for each of several business activities and is different for residents, interns, and non-U.S. physicians. Therefore, physicians should check with the DEA to make certain the proper registration is made. Two helpful booklets are the *United States Code of Federal Regulations, Title 21,* parts 1300 to end, revised April 1, 2001, which is available from the Office of the Federal Register, National Archives and Records Service, General Services Administration, and federal government bookstores, and *Physician's Manual,* 6th edition, available from the DEA, Office of Public Affairs, and regional DEA offices.

Record keeping and inventorying are required of physicians for the dispensing of narcotic and non-narcotic drugs to clients. The records must be kept for 2 years and are subject to DEA inspection. Inventory must be taken on the date of registration and every 2 years thereafter. The following is required:

1. Name, address, and DEA registration number
2. Date and time of inventory, that is, opening and closing of business
3. Signature of person(s) taking inventory
4. Inventory record to be on file for at least 2 years
5. Separate record required for schedule II drug

Security is necessary for controlled substances. These drugs must be kept in a locked or double-locked cabinet or a safe that is substantially constructed. Any loss is to be reported to the regional DEA office and local law enforcement.

Physicians who only prescribe narcotic or non-narcotic drugs are not required to keep the detailed record stated previously. State requirements differ, however, and may be more restrictive than federal requirements.

Drug Schedules

All controlled substances are divided into five schedules. A complete list should be obtained from a regional office of the DEA or can be found in the *United States Code of Federal Regulations, Title 21*. A brief summary is included in Box 4.1[2]

Issuing Prescriptions

According to the law, the only person authorized to issue prescriptions is the registrant. A prescription issued by the registrant may be communicated to the pharmacist by health care employees. This regulation may be less restrictive for medications not included in the Controlled Substances Act.

If the state requires triplicate prescription blanks, these will be used for prescribing drugs. These are not to be confused with the DEA form 224 described earlier. The triplicate blanks will be furnished by the state, and the regulations should be followed. For example, in some states, the triplicate blanks may be sequentially numbered.

All prescriptions for controlled substances must be dated and signed on the day issued, bearing the full name and address of the client and the name, address, and DEA registration number of the registrant. The prescription must be written in ink or typewritten and must be signed by hand by the physician or registrant.

Physicians must also know the laws of their state on controlled substances. The state regulations may be more strict than federal regulations and may require a separate state registration.

Narcotics laws should be studied carefully by any physician who opens an office. The *Code of Federal Regulations, Title 21,* mentioned earlier, should be obtained either via the Internet or from the nearest federal government bookstore and studied carefully before controlled substances are handled in the health care setting.

▲ CRITICAL THINKING EXERCISE

Identify medical specialty clinics that might dispense as well as prescribe controlled substances and discuss their usages.

IN THE NEWS

July 28, 2006, law enforcement authorities across the United States simultaneously arrested 31 members of Operation Somalia Express, a criminal organization that had a monopoly on U.S. khat drug distribution. The khat—5 tons worth $2 million—was destined for U.S. communities. Khat, cultivated daily in Kenya and Ethiopia, is a plant that contains cathinone, a stimulant classified as a Schedule I controlled substance. It is most potent when chewed within days of cultivation so the traffickers must operate efficiently to transport it from the Horn of Africa. According to the DEA, users of khat chew the leaves and young shoots of the plant, swallowing the juice and storing the residue in the side of the mouth until the cheeks bulge. The primary effects of chewing are euphoria and stimulation with numerous side effects including anorexia, heart disease, hypertension, and cancer of the mouth.

B O X 4.1 **Drugs Schedules**

Schedule I

This schedule lists drugs of high potential for abuse and that have no currently accepted medical use. Schedule I drugs can be used by physicians only for purposes of research, which must be approved by the Food and Drug Administration and the DEA, and only after a separate DEA registration as a researcher is obtained. The manufacture, importation, and sale of these drugs is prohibited.

Examples include heroin, marijuana, and lysergic acid diethylamide (LSD).

Schedule II

These drugs have current accepted medical use in the United States, but with severe restrictions. These drugs have a high potential of abuse that may lead to severe psychological or physical dependence.

Examples of schedule II narcotics include morphine, codeine, and oxycodone with aspirin (Percodan). Examples of non-narcotics include amphetamines, methylphenidate (Ritalin), and pentobarbital (Nembutal).

When these drugs are ordered, the physician must use a special order form that is preprinted with the physician's name and address. The form is issued in triplicate. One copy is kept in the physician's file. The remaining copies are forwarded to the supplier, who, after filling the order, keeps a copy and forwards the third copy to the nearest DEA office.

Prescription orders for schedule II drugs must be written and signed by the physician. Some states, by law, require special prescription blanks with more than one copy. The physician's registration number must appear on the blank. The order may not be telephoned in to the pharmacy except in an emergency, as defined by the DEA. A prescription for schedule II drugs may not be refilled.

Schedule III

These drugs have less potential for abuse than substances in schedules I and II. They have accepted medical use for treatment in the United States, but abuse may lead to moderate or low physical dependence or high psychological dependence.

Examples of schedule III narcotics include various drug combinations containing codeine and paregoric. Examples of non-narcotics include amphetamine-like compounds and secobarbital.

Schedule IV

These drugs have a lower potential for abuse than those in schedule III and have accepted medical use in the United States, but their abuse still may lead to limited physical or psychological dependence.

Examples include chloral hydrate, meprobamate, chlordiazepoxide (Librium), diazepam (Valium), and propoxyphene (Darvon).

Schedule III and IV drugs require either a written or oral prescription by the prescribing physician. If authorized by the physician on the initial prescription, the client may have the prescription refilled up to the number of refills authorized, which may not exceed five times or beyond 6 months from the date that the prescription was issued.

Schedule V

These drugs have less potential for abuse than drugs in schedule IV and their abuse may be limited to physical or psychological dependence. Refills are the same as for drugs in schedules III and IV.

Examples include cough medications containing codeine and antidiarrheals such as diphenoxylate/atropine (Lomotil).

Types of Court

As indicated earlier, the type of court that hears a particular case depends on the offense or complaint. In criminal cases, the type of court depends on the nature of the offense and where it occurs. In civil cases, it depends on the amount of money involved and where the parties reside. The jury and judge are neutral arbitrators of the evidence.

Courts also are classified as lower or higher, inferior or superior. A **lower** or **inferior court** has less authority than a **higher** or **superior court.**

Three jurisdictions belong only to federal courts: federal crimes, such as racketeering and bank robbery; constitutional issues; and civil action involving parties not living in the same state. Figure 4–4 illustrates the federal court system.

The U.S. Supreme Court is the highest court in the federal court system. Directly under the jurisdiction of the U.S. Supreme Court are the U.S. Court of Claims, the U.S. Court of Customs and Patent Office, and the U.S. Court of Appeals. The circuit courts direct the actions of the U.S. federal district courts and tax courts. In turn, the U.S. Supreme Court directs the actions of all courts: federal, state, trial, and appellate.

The pattern for state courts is similar to the pattern for federal courts. There are inferior or lower courts and a process of appeals. Figure 4–5 illustrates the state court system. The lower courts hear cases involving civil matters, small claims, housing, traffic, and some misdemeanors. The State Superior Court has general jurisdiction in all types of civil and criminal cases. The **court of appeals** has power to review decisions of this court. The court of appeals may reverse, remand, modify, or affirm a decision of a lower court. The final route of appeal is to the State Supreme Court, the determination of which becomes the law of the state.

Each state defines by statute the types of cases a particular court will hear and the maximum money value of the cases over which it has jurisdiction. In the event litigation does arise in a civil matter, physicians and their health care employees will most likely find themselves in a state court. Other civil matters may also take place in probate court and small claims court.

Probate Court

Probate law oversees the distribution of a person's estate upon death. In **probate court** (sometimes called **estate court**), the physician may decide to initiate action on the collection of a bill owed by a deceased client. Generally, the health care employee represents the interests of the physician and attempts to locate the responsible person or party for the debt, whose name can be obtained from the deceased client's family or lawyer, from the hospital, or from the mortuary. If unable to obtain a name from these sources, the health care employee must write or call the county seat in which the estate is being settled. The county probate court recorder will provide information concerning the filing of the claim (in court, to the executor of the estate, or elsewhere), the proper forms to file, and when the claim must be submitted. Quick action is required because most states have a file period of from 4 to 12 months after the publication of notice in a newspaper by the administrator or executor (Fig. 4–6).

Once the probate forms are ready to be mailed, the health care employee sends them by certified mail, return receipt requested. This establishes that the documents were received and by whom. The administrator will either accept or reject the claim. If it is accepted, payment will follow, but it may be delayed for months in the courts. If it is rejected and the physician believes the bill is justified, a lawsuit may be filed against the administrator within

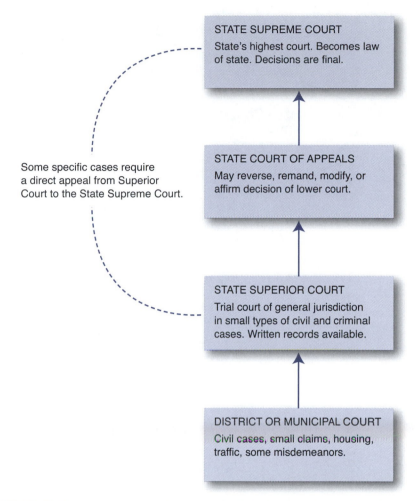

FIGURE 4-5 Titles of courts vary from state to state, but this diagram illustrates the overall structure of the court system in most states.

a designated amount of time, depending on the state. Health care employees should be aware of their particular state's time limits.

Keep in mind that even though you may be hesitant to collect a deceased client's bill, the physician rendered services for the client and deserves payment. Failure to file a claim may be construed by others as an admission of poor medical care on the part of the physician.

Small Claims Court

Small claims court allows the physician or physician representative to file action against a client for an unpaid or delinquent account. In the state of Virginia, for example, small claims court has jurisdiction over cases when the plaintiff seeks monetary judgment up to $2000. In addition to the judgment of the amount owed, the physician plaintiff may also recover the costs of the suit. There is no representation by attorney. The plaintiff bringing the action files a preprinted form identifying facts in the account to be collected. A **summons** is issued on the complaint requesting the appearance of the defendant before the judge.

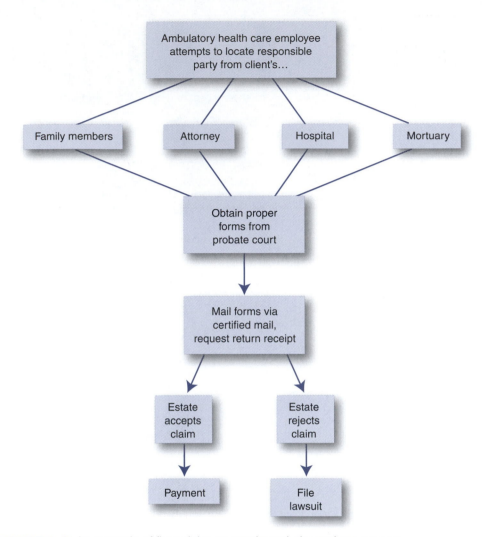

FIGURE 4–6 An example of financial recovery through the probate process.

The defendant is given time to file a cross-complaint against the plaintiff for any possible grievance the defendant may have. A date is set for delivery and decision.

The plaintiff presents the facts in the case, and the defendant responds to the allegations or charges. Both parties may **subpoena** witnesses to testify on their behalf. After all information is heard, the matter goes to the judge for a decision. If judgment is in favor of the defendant, there is no right to appeal. However, if judgment is in favor of the plaintiff, the defendant may appeal the decision to a higher court.

The prudent health care employee will contact the clerk of the small claims court for instructions and information regarding the procedures to follow. This is in direct contrast to lawsuits in higher courts, where court clerks cannot assist the parties in completing forms.

▲ CRITICAL THINKING EXERCISE

Although probate court and small claims court are avenues to collect a client's account, discuss the disadvantages of doing so.

IN THE NEWS

The City and County of Denver, Colorado stated in a February 2006 news release that they were offering "convenient, walk-in lunch hour clinics throughout the year to help answer your small claims and collection questions." The clinics were 2-hour sessions with volunteer attorneys to provide small claim procedural information. Civil Division staff hosted the collection clinics to provide tips on how to collect judgments. Does your state offer these services?

Subpoenas

Physicians may find themselves in court even though they and their employees have practiced good preventive measures. No matter what the dispute or reason for **litigation,** physicians need to be adequately prepared. The reasons for court appearances are numerous, but most commonly the physician will be a defendant, a witness, or an **expert witness (medical)** in civil or criminal trials; in sanity and probate contests; in personal injury actions; or in cases arising under insurance policies including life, health, or accident.

In any of these cases, physicians may appear with or without a subpoena. A subpoena is an order commanding attendance in a specific court or office, at a specific time, under penalty for failure to do so unless a protective order from the court invalidates the requirement. The subpoena may be signed by the clerk of the court, a notary public, or an attorney. The subpoena may require a **deposition** to be taken rather than an actual appearance in court.

The attendance requested in a subpoena may be of a person (physician or health care employee) or of data (medical record). The latter is a ***subpoena duces tecum,*** which requires the witness to appear and to bring certain records. The physician most likely would not need to appear to identify a record; proper identification usually can be done by an employee. The physician would be required, however, if the record needed to be interpreted.

A **court order** is an order issued only by a judge to appear or to request certain records. The release of any records requested in a court order does not require the client's permission. Any records related to substance abuse, mental health, or dangerous communicable diseases also require a court order. State laws differ on rules related to court orders but generally these orders have stronger force of the law than a summons, a subpoena, or a *subpoena duces tecum.*

Whether a subpoena or a court order, it should authorize witness fees, photocopying fees, or mileage fees. If fees are not authorized, they are to be requested when the subpoena is served. If the physician is being subpoenaed, the subpoena must be hand-delivered to the physician. However, because so many subpoenas are served and there are so few officers to serve them, some subpoenas may be served to the physician's employee instead of to the physician. In such cases, the physician, out of courtesy, appears in court as though the subpoena was served by an officer to him or her. If the medical record is subpoenaed, the subpoena may be served to an employee. Any questions about a subpoena or its circumstances should be taken to an attorney immediately.

The Trial Process

A case may be tried before a judge or a judge and jury. Usually, trial courts have a jury, but the parties to a trial may waive (voluntarily give up) their right to a jury trial.

First, the jury, consisting of 6 to 12 people, must be selected (Fig. 4–7). A pool of potential jurors is chosen at random from voter registration lists and auto license records in the area. How the actual jurors are picked from this pool depends on the level of court, the type of case being tried, and local court rules. Once the jurors are selected, they are given the oath by a clerk or judge.

The trial procedure then begins. **Opening statements** usually are made by each attorney, first for the plaintiff and then for the defendant. Such statements outline the facts each party hopes to establish during the trial. The plaintiff's attorney calls the first witness and asks questions **(examination of witness).** This part of the process is called **direct examination.** The defendant's attorney then cross-examines the witness **(cross-examination).** This procedure continues until the plaintiff's entire case has been presented. The case for the defense is presented in the same manner. The direct examinations and cross-examinations recur. In a criminal case, the state must prove guilt "beyond a reasonable doubt," whereas in a civil case it is by a preponderance of evidence. Then both attorneys rest their cases, that is, indicate that no further evidence or testimony is to be given.

If it is a jury trial, the judge then instructs the jury on the law governing the case. The attorney for each party is allowed **closing arguments,** after which the judge charges the jury to reach a fair verdict based on the evidence presented. Then the jury is ushered from the courtroom to consider the case and reach a verdict.

In civil court, the judge or jury finds for the plaintiff or for the defendant. If the verdict is found in favor of the defendant, the case is dismissed. If the plaintiff wins the case, a monetary settlement usually is awarded, the amount determined by the judge or jury.

In a criminal trial, if the defendant is found guilty, the judge imposes sentence. At sentencing, the court can commit the defendant to an institution or allow probation. At the end of the trial, the judge informs the defendant of all rights to appeal. If the defendant is found not guilty, the case is dismissed.

Expert Witness

In medical cases, an expert witness is a person specifically qualified in medicine who can testify in court as to what the professional standard of care is in the same or a similar community. An expert witness is necessary if the subject of the court action is beyond the general understanding of the average layperson or if the knowledge of the expert witness will aid in discovering the truth. Refer to the vignette "Can She Be an Expert Witness" at the beginning of the chapter.

As expert witnesses, physicians testify as to what they see, hear, know to be fact, and is the recognized standard of care. Opinions not based on their experience or expertise, certain out-of-court statements, and conclusions are not admissible in most cases. Expert

FIGURE 4–7 Graphical representation of a jury.

witnesses in medical cases are usually skilled in the art, science, or profession of medicine and may be practicing medicine or teaching in a school of medicine. In litigation, attorneys may have difficulty obtaining an expert witness who is geographically close because experts are often hesitant to testify about a situation that may appear to contradict their own peers.

Expert witnesses are expected to be reputable, honest, and impartial. The attorney who has called the witness will try to establish the witness's training, experience, intelligence, and accuracy. Witnesses should talk in lay terms rather than medical language and bear in mind that their dress and appearance may influence the judge and jury. Attorneys cannot prompt or cue witnesses.

Expert witnesses may wish to illustrate or clarify their testimony by employing visual aids such as electronic media, photographs, diagrams, charts, radiographs, skeletons, and human-type models. In some instances, sketch artists or illustrators may be employed. During cross-examination, witnesses may face difficulties. The cross-examining attorney may try to intimidate the witness or create confusion. Witnesses should take their time and answer truthfully. They should not be afraid to say, "I don't know," if that is the case.

Expert witnesses are entitled to a fee commensurate with their time away from their practice or teaching for the case, their preparation for the case, and their participation in the case. If questioned during cross-examination regarding a fee for witnessing, they should answer truthfully. A fee should be established before serving as an expert witness rather than on a contingency basis.

If a health care employee or a physician is subpoenaed to be an expert witness, legal counsel should be sought. Ethically such testimony should not be seen as adversarial to peers. An attorney will guide, advise, and take whatever legal action is indicated.

We cannot overstress how important legal counsel is in the case of any questions or doubts. Physicians often seek consultation on difficult medical problems and should do no less for themselves and their employees if faced with litigation.

Summary

This introduction to law does not attempt to provide all the necessary information the health care employee may need. It provides basic information, not legal advice. However, ambulatory health care employees must be knowledgeable of the law and aware of their professional responsibilities so that they can act responsibly. Many activities in health care require knowledge of the law to prevent illegal acts; however, when in doubt always seek legal counsel.

IN THE NEWS

Numerous websites feature companies, many of them legal firms, that provide medical expert witnesses. One such company details their services. An expert witness will:

1. Gather data and review all available records including hospital and physician medical records, x-rays, depositions, affidavits, and other pertinent data to compare what actually happened against the standard of care.
2. Provide a signed opinion letter if there has been a deviation from the standard of care.
3. Provide continuing support through discovery, deposition, and trail testimony.

QUESTIONS FOR REVIEW

1. Name and describe the three branches of the federal government.

_____

_____

2. Define the two basic types of law and their development.

_____

_____

3. Describe civil and criminal law and give an example of each.

_____

_____

4. Explain the Controlled Substances Act.

_____

_____

5. List the differences between Schedule I and Schedule V drugs.

_____

_____

6. The importance of accuracy in registering, record keeping, and security of controlled substances is necessary because

_____

_____

7. Describe the differences between a lower and a higher court.

_____

_____

8. Define probate court and describe how a health care provider might need to use one.

_____

_____

9. Define small claims court and name a situation in which a health care provider might use one.

_____

_____

10. Compare and contrast the difference among a subpoena, a *subpoena duces tecum,* and a *court order.*

_____

_____

11. Summarize the trial process with a judge and a jury.

_____

_____

12. Explain why an expert witness might be used.

_____

_____

CLASSROOM EXERCISES

1. Describe a situation in which an understanding of the law is important to a medical receptionist.

2. If you were involved in a civil case, describe the process the case would follow and identify the factors that would determine the appropriate court.

3. Compare and contrast a summons, a subpoena, and court order. Give an example of the use of each.

4. A physician from another state is coming into your established practice. What must be done about narcotics registration?

5. Discuss the relevance of any cases currently under consideration in the U.S. Supreme Court that directly affect the health care employee.

6. In the vignette at the beginning of the chapter, "Can She Be an Expert Witness?", what issues does the medical assistant educator consider?

7. Clarence calls requesting a refill for Percodan. Your records show that he has not been seen by the physician for almost 1 year. The doctor is away from the office for 1 week. What will you do? Consider the legal implications.

REFERENCES

1. Drug Enforcement Administration: Physician's Manual. U.S. Department of Justice, Washington, DC, 1990.
2. Code of Federal Regulation, No. 12, Parts 1300 to end. Office of Federal Registrar, Washington, DC, 1991.

WEB RESOURCES

▲ Drug Enforcement Administration. www.dea.gov
▲ Office of Diversion Control. www.deadiversion.usdoj.gov/index.html
▲ Physician's News Digest. www.physiciansnews.com/law

CHAPTER 5

Regulations and Professional Liability for Health Professionals

> " *When you get right down to the root of the meaning of the word 'succeed,' you find it simply means to follow through.* "
>
> F. W. Nichol

KEY TERMS

agent An agent is a person (the health care employee) appointed by a principal party (the physician or provider) to perform authorized acts in the name and under the control and direction of the principal.

alternative dispute resolution (ADR) Methods outside the judicial system used to solve potential malpractice actions; methods include arbitration and mediation.

assault Assault refers to a threat to inflict injury with an apparent ability to do so.

battery Battery is the unlawful touching, beating, or laying hold of persons or their clothing without consent.

breach of contract Failure to comply with the terms of a valid contract.

defamation Spoken or written words concerning someone that tend to injure that person's reputation and for which damages can be recovered. Two types of defamation are libel, which is false, defamatory writing, such as published material, effigy, or picture; and slander, which is false, malicious, defamatory spoken words.

malfeasance Commission of an unlawful act.

medical malpractice Professional negligence of physicians or providers.

misfeasance Improper performance of an act resulting in injury to another.

negligence (medical) Doing some act that a reasonable and prudent physician or provider would not do or failing to do some act that a reasonable and prudent physician or provider would do.

nonfeasance Failure to perform an act when there is a duty to do so.

protected health information (PHI) All the past, present, and future physical and mental conditions of an individual's health care.

res ipsa loquitur A Latin phrase meaning "the thing speaks for itself." A doctrine of negligence law.

respondeat superior A Latin phrase meaning "let the master answer;" that is, the provider or physician is responsible for employee acts.

summons An order, in a civil case, from the court directing the sheriff or other appropriate official to notify the defendant where and when to appear.

tickler file A periodic reminder to do specific tasks on schedule; usually daily, weekly, or monthly.

tort Wrongful act committed by one person against another person or against property; distinguished from a breach of contract.

LEARNING OBJECTIVES

Upon successful completion of this chapter, you will be able to:

1. Define key terms.
2. Identify four common requirements for a physician to be licensed.
3. Identify three conditions under which a physician's license may be revoked.
4. Explain professional liability for physicians.
5. Discuss the meaning of standard of care.
6. Discuss confidentiality as related to the standard of care.
7. Summarize the key points of HIPAA related to health care.
8. List three elements necessary for a contract to be valid.
9. Compare and contrast intentional and unintentional torts.
10. Identify the four Ds of negligence for physicians.
11. Discuss *res ipsa loquitur* and *respondeat superior*.
12. Explain the term *statute of limitations* and identify the three most common points for injury-related statute of limitations to begin.
13. Restate, in your own words, the importance of professional liability insurance.
14. Recall ten guidelines for risk management.

Vignette: Who has a right to know?

Kelly, a first-year medical assistant student, tells her instructor that she thinks she may be pregnant and wonders what she should do. The instructor recommends that Kelly go to the campus health center for a pregnancy test. When Kelly's test is positive, she again discusses her case with her instructor. As a single woman, Kelly decides she cannot support a child now but is not sure whether to have the baby and put it up for adoption or to have an abortion. After a few days and a discussion with the father of the child, their decision is to have an abortion.

Kelly returns to the campus health clinic for her test results so that she can take them to the abortion clinic. The certified medical assistant, a former graduate of the school's medical assistant program and a health center employee, refuses to give Kelly the test results, saying, "You'll have to talk to the nurse practitioner. I don't believe in abortion." The nurse practitioner gives her the laboratory results.

Without an understanding of laws that directly relate to physicians, health care employee may inadvertently cause difficulties. Therefore it is important to consider those laws and regulations that directly influence the actions of health care employees and physicians. The law is, at times, both complicated and vague. This book cannot cover all parts of the law as it may affect physicians and employees. Only laws related to the practice of medicine in an office or clinic are emphasized.

One of the greatest fears of employees and physicians is the threat of litigation. Caring for persons who may be ill, apprehensive, in pain, or suffering from a life-threatening condition is risky. Such a risk carries the possibility of litigation, which becomes a reality when a **summons** is served on the physician or when someone is subpoenaed to testify in court.

Litigation may be sought for many reasons. A client may sue the physician for **negligence (medical).** Perhaps a contractual arrangement has been violated (**breach of contract**) or a **tort** has been committed.

Medical Practice Acts

Medical practice acts are state statutes that define the practice of medicine, describe methods of licensure, and set guidelines for suspension or revocation of a license. All 50 states have such statutes to protect their citizens from harm by unqualified persons practicing medicine.

Licensure

Physicians must be licensed to practice medicine in the United States. States differ in their licensing requirements. The more common requirements include graduation from an accredited medical school, completion of an internship, and successful completion of the United States Medical Licensing Examination (USMLE), which was implemented in 1994. Non-U.S.-trained and non-U.S.-educated physicians are required to pass the USMLE before being allowed to practice in the United States.

Physicians who choose to practice in more than one state must satisfy the license requirements of each state. This may be done by requiring physicians to meet each state's endorsement requirements.

Many states require a complete and unrestricted license to provide medical services. The Department of Defense is encouraging states to require full licensure of its military personnel. Physicians engaging strictly in research and not practicing medicine need not have a license in some states.

License Renewal

Physicians renew their licenses periodically, and payment of a fee is usually required. The physician receives notice at the time of renewal. Documentation of continuing medical education (CME) is commonly a requirement for renewal; however, some states only require payment of a fee. Specific state requirements differ. Appropriate credits are identified in the state statutes and may include (1) reading of books, papers, and publications; (2) teaching health professionals; (3) attending approved courses, workshops, and seminars; and (4) self-instruction.[1]

Employees may be responsible for keeping records of the physician's continuing medical education activities. To do so, they must have the state's requirements on file and be able to verify the credits as required.

License Revocation and Suspension

A physician's license to practice may be revoked or suspended as a result of (1) conviction of a crime, (2) unprofessional conduct, and (3) personal or professional incapacity. Each of these conditions is defined by state statute.

Conviction of a crime is a more obvious reason for license revocation than is unprofessional conduct or personal or professional incapacity. Examples include physicians who are convicted of child abuse or commit sexual assault against clients. Unprofessional conduct of all licensed health care professionals, including physicians, generally is defined by law. Although these acts may not be crimes, such conduct is unacceptable according to state law and therefore is punishable. Examples of unprofessional conduct include falsifying any records regarding licensing, being dishonest, and impersonating another physician. Personal or professional incapacity includes chronic substance abuse, continuing to practice when severe physical limitations prevent adequate care, and practicing outside the scope of training.

Usually charges against physicians are made by the physicians' licensing board in all three conditions necessitating the suspension or revocation of a physician's license. In all states, the basic procedure for disciplinary action is similar. Most boards are required to give the physician licensee sufficient notice of the charges and allow the physician legal counsel and a hearing. The board then investigates, prosecutes, makes a judgment, and sentences. Some states have empowered their licensing boards to suspend a license to practice on a temporary basis without a hearing when the physician poses an immediate threat. In other words, no due process is necessary if the physician poses an immediate threat.

Professional Liability

Once physicians become licensed, they become legally liable for their actions as physicians. They are responsible, accountable, obligated, and legally bound by law. Their liability can be either civil or criminal or both. Criminal liability is less common in ambulatory health care than civil liability. Criminal liability results when an individual commits an act that is considered to be an offense against society as a whole. The legal term **malfeasance** reflects this liability. Malfeasance is the commission of an unlawful act.

Examples of criminal liability for the physician include fraud in insurance billing, committing child abuse, and the evasion or breach of the Controlled Substances Act. Physicians found to be grossly negligent or reckless in the death of a client may be held criminally responsible. In some states, the failure of physicians to make certain reports (e.g., child or elder abuse) required by law may be a crime.

Civil liability identifies conflicts between individuals, corporations, government bodies, and other organizations. Examples of civil liability include tort and breach of contract. For example, civil liability occurs when the physician prescribes a pain medication over the phone for a migraine-like headache, not recalling that this person is recovering from hepatitis. Since the pain medication is contraindicated in hepatitis, the person becomes violently ill with resultant liver damage. In this example, **misfeasance** is the term used to describe the improper performance of an act that results in an injury to another.

Standard of Care

One cannot fully understand liability without some knowledge of standard of care principles. Acceptable standard of care requires that physicians use the ordinary and reasonable skill that would be commonly used by other reputable practitioners when caring for individuals. They are expected to perform those acts that a reasonable and prudent physician would perform. Failure to perform an act when there is a duty to do so is known as **nonfeasance.** The standard also dictates that physicians must not perform any acts that a reasonable and prudent physician would not perform. Physicians should always practice in the realm of safety and secure all necessary data on which to base a sound judgment. This includes obtaining a thorough medical history, a complete physical examination, and necessary laboratory tests. Physicians are expected to know what new therapeutic developments might benefit those in their care and still not subject them to undue risk.

Employees in health care also must adhere to a standard of care. The standard health care employee will be measured against depends on the task the employee is undertaking; the education, training, and experience of the employee; and the responsibility the physician has given the employee. For example, if the health care employee makes a diagnosis or treats a client, the employee could be held to the standard of care as the physician. If the employee is acting outside his or her level of competency and the client is injured as a result, the employee could be found negligent. Health care employees often act in a variety of roles, and they must understand the standard to which they could be held. If, on the other hand, the health care employee is mopping the floor, he or she will be held to the reasonable person standard of a custodial person rather than the standard of a specific health care professional.

The Health Insurance Portability and Accountability Act (HIPAA)

The Health Insurance Portability and Accountability Act (HIPAA) was passed by Congress in 1996 and applies to employer-based and commercially issued group health insurance. HIPAA requires (1) standardization of electronic patient health data, administrative data, and financial data; (2) unique health identifiers for individuals, employees, health plans, and health care providers; and (3) security standards to protect the confidentiality and integrity of the individually identifiable health information, past, present, or future.

Congress further required the Department of Health and Human Services (HHS) to develop privacy standards in order to protect health information. *The Privacy Rule* required all "covered entities" to protect and secure electronic data information by April 2003. The rule applies to **protected health information** (PHI) that is all the past, present, and future physical and mental conditions of an individual's health care. Under HIPAA, patients must grant written consent or permission to provide or disclose their PHI for any health care reason. Physicians must provide patients with a notice of their privacy practices that must include the right to:

▲ Restrict usage of PHI
▲ Request confidential communication
▲ Inspect and obtain a copy of the PHI
▲ Request any amendment to the PHI
▲ Receive an accounting of PHI disclosures

This is just a brief introduction of HIPAA regulations. Criminal penalties can be levied for noncompliance of the security standards of $100 per violation up to $25,000 per person for all identical violations in a calendar year. Knowingly obtaining or disclosing individually identifiable health information warrants a fine of $50,000 and imprisonment for 1 year. Watch for the HIPAA icon throughout the text for additional HIPAA applications.

Confidentiality

One of the main purposes of HIPAA is to ensure and protect a client's privacy related to health care issues. **REMEMBER...** Unless otherwise required by law, physicians must keep confidential any communication necessary to treatment of the client. The client's privacy must be protected. Physicians and their employees must be extremely careful that all infor-

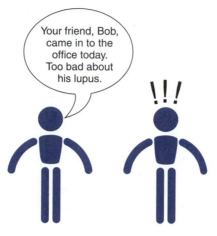

Confidentiality

FIGURE 5–1 An example of a breach of confidentiality.

mation gained through the care of the client is kept confidential and given only to those health professionals who have a medical need to know. Care should also be taken that any information communicated about a client cannot be overheard by others (Fig. 5–1).

In many cases, HIPAA regulations have meant that clinics reconsidered how clients are greeted, how basic personal information is viewed, how billing is discussed, how clients are addressed in the reception area and any other areas when personal information may be seen or heard. For example, a clinic that had a very open reception area created a cubicle at one side of their reception where private information is exchanged. Another clinic chooses to enclose their reception area in glass. No telephone calls are made to remind clients of their appointments or to discuss bills or laboratory results where any other party can hear. It is imperative that clients' charts or any personal information be out of view of others.

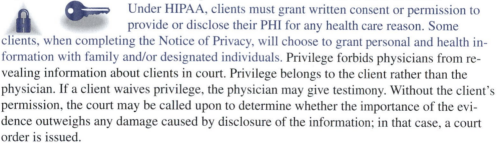 Under HIPAA, clients must grant written consent or permission to provide or disclose their PHI for any health care reason. Some clients, when completing the Notice of Privacy, will choose to grant personal and health information with family and/or designated individuals. Privilege forbids physicians from revealing information about clients in court. Privilege belongs to the client rather than the physician. If a client waives privilege, the physician may give testimony. Without the client's permission, the court may be called upon to determine whether the importance of the evidence outweighs any damage caused by disclosure of the information; in that case, a court order is issued.

Special consideration is given to the confidential nature of information about clients who test positive for HIV or have AIDS. All 50 states require reporting of AIDS cases, without the client's consent, to the Centers for Disease Control and Prevention or to their state's health department. Most physicians would inform their clients of this notification requirement as a matter of courtesy. States have adopted a variety of legislation about disclosure of confidential information regarding HIV and AIDS. Check in your particular state for detailed information. Additional protection is also given to clients who seek treatment for mental health or substance abuse issues. When in doubt, seek legal advice.

▲ CRITICAL THINKING EXERCISE

To become HIPAA compliant, how do you protect confidentiality when the office area is in the hallway of a medical facility or when the reception area is very open?

In your podiatrist's office, they have a sign-in sheet requesting your name, phone number, insurance number, and social security number. What do you do?

Contracts

Health care professionals are liable for negligence issues and contract principles. A physician–client relationship or contract is normally a prerequisite for litigation against a physician. This is known as *contract law*. A breach of a contract can bring litigation against a physician. A tort may occur, which is a wrongful act or injury committed by one person against another person (not related to a contract) and for which the court will provide a remedy.

Health care employees and their physicians are parties to contracts on a daily basis. When a physician accepts a client, a contract has been made. When the office assistant calls an office supply company to reorder office stationery, the assistant acts as the physician's **agent** in making a contract.

For a contract to be valid, it must be an agreement between two or more competent people to do or not to do a certain task for payment or for the rendering of a benefit, and the agreement must be lawful.

An example in health care occurs when a client calls the office to make an appointment for an annual physical examination. Assuming that the physician is a bona fide physician and the client is a competent adult, the first two parts of the contract exist. The performance of a physical examination is a lawful act, so part three of the contract exists. The client is given a statement of the charges, and the fee is paid. Hence, the contract is valid in all respects (Fig. 5–2).

A contract can be expressed or implied. An expressed contract can be written or oral, but all facets of the contract must be specifically stated and understood. An oral contract is as legally binding as a written one; however, it may be more difficult to prove. Physicians' telephone contacts with clients are examples of oral contracts, especially when medical advice is given. A written contract requires that all necessary aspects of the agreement be in writing. Each state, in its statute of frauds, identifies those contracts that must be in writing. Usually included in this list are deeds and mortgages. Most states' statute of frauds includes a section that is pertinent to health care, that is, an agreement made by a third party to pay for the medical expenses of another. Such an agreement has to be in writing to be valid. If Elaine tells the medical receptionist that she will pay the medical expenses for her good friend, Diane, the receptionist should ask Elaine to fill out a form to that

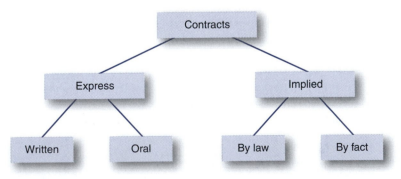

FIGURE 5–2 Contracts, either expressed or implied, can be legally binding.

effect and affix her signature to it. If not properly executed, it may be impossible to collect the bill.

Implied contracts are the most common form of contracts occurring in health care. Such contracts occur every time the physician and client discuss what course of treatment to take and an agreement is reached. An implied agreement does not require a specific expression of the parties involved but is still valid if all points of the contract exist. An implied contract may be implied from the facts or circumstances of the situation or by the law. When a client complains of a sore throat and the physician does a throat culture to diagnose and treat the ailment, a contract is implied by the circumstances of the situation. A contract implied by the law is seen in the example of the physician who administers epinephrine after a client has gone into anaphylactic shock. The law will say that the physician did what the client would have requested had there been an expressed agreement.

Contracts made by the mentally incompetent, the legally insane, those under heavy influence of drugs or alcohol, infants, and some minors are not valid. Such persons are not considered by the law to be competent to enter into binding contracts.

REMEMBER... Health care employees are generally considered agents of their physician-employer. An agent is a person (the health care employee) appointed by a principal party (the physician) to perform authorized acts in the name and under the control and direction of the principal. As agents, health care employees must be careful of their actions, which could become binding on their physicians. For example, an employee might promise a cure that in fact is not possible.

The physician's fiduciary obligation, posed by their professional ethics, causes courts to look outside the parameters of contract law when determining the physician's obligation to treat a client. Health care professionals are constrained in their ability to withdraw from contractual relationships by judicial case law, which has rules against patient abandonment.

Abandonment

Once the physician–client relationship has been established, physicians can be found liable if they abandon their clients. To avoid charges of abandonment, the physician should withdraw formally from a case or discharge a client formally. This requires giving reasonable notice to the client with the recommendation for the client to seek further medical care. The notice should be sent so that the client has ample time to secure another physician.

A physician may wish to withdraw from the case if the client fails to follow instructions, take the prescribed medications, or return for recommended appointments. To withdraw formally from a case, a physician should notify the client in writing, state the reasons for the dismissal, and to indicate a future date when the physician is no longer responsible. Such a letter should be sent by certified mail with a return receipt requested. Figure 5–3 shows an example of a letter of withdrawal. A copy of the letter and the returned receipt are kept in the client's file. To further protect a physician from abandonment charges, all canceled and missed appointments should be noted on the client's chart.

Breach of Contract

A breach of contract arises when one of the parties involved fails to meet the contractual components. For example, the contract may be violated when the client does not pay the bill or refuses to follow medical advice. The contract can be breached when the physician fails to use the treatment promised, promises to do a procedure and then allows someone else to do the procedure, or promises a cure and no cure results. Such breaches of contract are cause for litigation in which the court attempts to make reimbursement to the client for losses suffered. Usually this reimbursement is in the form of a monetary award.

RECOMMENDED TERMINATION LETTER

Letter of Withdrawal from a Case

Dear_____ :

I find it necessary to inform you that I am withdrawing from further professional attendance upon you for the reason that you have persisted in refusing to follow my medical advice and treatment. Since your condition requires medical attention, I suggest that you place yourself under the care of another physician without delay. If you so desire, I shall be available to attend you for a reasonable time after you have received this letter, but in no event for more than five days.

This should give you ample time to select a physician of your choice from the many competent physicians in this city. With your approval, I will make available to this physician your case history and information regarding the diagnosis and treatment you have received from me.

Very truly yours,

_____ M.D.

FIGURE 5–3 Letter of withdrawal. © 2003 Professional Management & Marketing.

Torts

Tort law is the area of law health care professionals are involved in because it identifies negligence and **medical malpractice.** Health care employees or physicians may commit a tort that may result in litigation.

A tort is a wrongful act committed by one person against another person or against property that causes harm to that person or property. A tort results if there is damage or injury to the client proximately caused by the conduct of the physician or the health care employee that does not meet the standard of care governing either the physician or the health care employee.

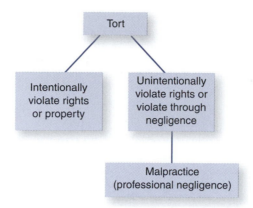

FIGURE 5–4 Torts are violations, either intentional or unintentional.

If a physician commits a wrongful act against a client with no resultant client harm, a tort has not been committed.

The two main classifications of torts are intentional and unintentional/negligence acts. Intentional torts or wrongs involve the intentional commission of a violation of another person's rights. Unintentional or negligent wrongs may be the result of the omission or the commission of an act. Malpractice is an unintentional tort (Fig. 5–4). It is a specific type of negligence that occurs when the standard of care commonly expected from health care professionals is not met. It is also known as professional negligence.

Vignette: Focus on Clients
CAN'T I TELL MY FRIEND?

To continue with the dilemma of Kelly's pregnancy in "Who Has a Right To Know?" consider the following information.

Several days later in the medical assistant clinical class, another medical assistant instructor overhears Nancy, a student who is receiving work experience in the campus health center, breach a confidence and tell other students in the class about Kelly's pregnancy and abortion.

The program's coordinator privately speaks with Nancy about the breach of confidentiality. Nancy responds, "I didn't tell the whole class. I only told my friend."

Professional Negligence or Malpractice

Failure to perform professional duties according to the accepted standard of care is negligence. More specifically, negligence is performing an act that a reasonable and prudent physician would not perform or the failure to perform an act that a reasonable and prudent physician would perform. Professional negligence, as defined previously, is the same as malpractice. Malpractice may be described as professional negligence.

Professional negligence is more easily prevented than defended. Obviously, physicians do not wish to be found negligent or become involved in a malpractice suit of any kind. However, consumers are more aware of their rights today than ever before. Therefore physicians must protect the physician–client relationship at all times and be above reproach in the performance of their duties.

The Four Ds of Negligence

The four Ds of negligence are duty, derelict, direct cause, and damages:

1. *Duty* exists when the physician–client relationship has been established. For example, the client calls the office to make an appointment, keeps the appointment, and makes another to return for further treatment.
2. *Derelict* is more difficult to define. The client must prove that the physician failed to comply with the standards required and dictated by the profession.
3. *Direct cause* implies that any damage or injuries that resulted from the physician's breach of duty were directly related to that breach and that no intermittent circumstances or intervening acts could have caused the damages.
4. *Damages* refers to the compensation provided for injuries suffered by the client. The most common in medical professional liability cases is monetary compensation, which may be actual, or compensatory damages and exemplary or punitive damages. Actual damages are those that compensate the client for injuries sustained and nothing more. These include past medical care, loss of wages, and future medical care. Exemplary or punitive damages are compensation that punishes the defendant and awards the client for pain, suffering, and mental anguish. Punitive damages may be limited by law in some states.

Vignette: Who is responsible?

Mrs. Farley had a tubal ligation. She was informed of the risks and signed consent forms before surgery. Five months later she returned to the same physician, who determined that she was pregnant. After the birth of Mrs. Farley's baby, the attending physician examined both of her fallopian tubes and found that one was ligated, but the other appeared normal. Mrs. Farley sued the physician who performed the tubal ligation on the basis of res ipsa loquitur.

OUTCOME: The court held that Mrs. Farley could not rely on the doctrine of res ipsa loquitur to establish the medical malpractice claim against the physician. The court held that "the doctrine of res ipsa loquitur cannot be invoked where the existence of negligence is wholly a matter of conjecture and the circumstances are not proved, but must themselves be presumed, or when it may be inferred that there was no negligence on the part of the defendant." The doctrine only holds in cases in which the defendant's negligence is the only inference that can reasonably and legitimately be drawn from the circumstances. This was not the case here. The court stated that this was probably one of those cases in which the sterilization procedure failed; the ligation was performed, but the ligation band came off soon thereafter.

FARLEY V MEADOWS, 404 SE2D 537 (1991).

Res Ipsa Loquitur

The doctrine of **res ipsa loquitur,** "the thing speaks for itself," is a rule of law of negligence. It relates chiefly to cases of foreign bodies being left in clients and instruments slipping during surgical procedures, burns from heating modalities, and injury to a portion of the client's body outside the field of treatment. In other words, the negligence is obvious; the result was such that it could not have occurred without someone being negligent.

Intentional Torts

Intentional torts are intentional acts violating another person's rights or property. The ethical obligation to "do no harm" to a client *(nonfeasance)*

is the basis for any intentional tort action. If the principle of nonfeasance were never violated and there was no harm to the client there could be no grounds for lawsuits based on intentional torts.

Some of the more common intentional torts likely to occur in ambulatory health care are **assault** and **battery**, **defamation**, and invasion of privacy. Assault and battery are terms often used together, however, assault rarely occurs in the medical setting. Assault refers to a threat to inflict injury with an apparent ability to do so. Battery, in the medical context, occurs when a client receives treatment without having given consent to do so; it is the unlawful touching, beating, or laying hold of persons or their clothing without consent. Some intentional torts such as assault and battery may also violate criminal laws and can become complaints in both criminal court and civil court. In this situation, separate trials will be held, one civil and one criminal. Recall from Chapter 4 that in a civil case the plaintiff must show, by a preponderance of evidence, that a tort has been committed, whereas in a criminal case the prosecution must prove its case beyond a reasonable doubt.

When a battery occurs, an individual's right has been invaded. Individuals have the right to be free from invasion of their persons. Regardless of whether the procedure constituting the battery improves the client's health, the client must consent to the treatment.

Defamation is spoken or written words that tend to injure a person's reputation and for which damages can be recovered. One type of defamation is libel, which is false, malicious, defamatory writing, such as published material, effigies, and pictures. Another type of defamation is slander, which is the false and malicious defamatory spoken word. For defamation to be a tort, a third person must hear or see the slander or libel and understand it.

Invasion of privacy is the unauthorized publicity of client information. Medical records and treatments cannot be released without the client's knowledge and permission. Clients have the right to be left alone and the right to be free from unwanted publicity and exposure to public view.

Torts can be prevented by practicing legally and ethically. The standard of care in the health care setting needs to be excellent. The privacy of clients must be guarded, their bodies and possessions must be respected, and their reputations must be protected. The rights of clients are to be protected by all who come in contact with them.

Doctrine of *Respondeat Superior*

Professional liability exists for both employer and employee. Physicians are responsible not only for their own actions of negligence but also for the negligent actions of their employees under the doctrine of *respondeat superior.* This Latin phrase means "let the master answer." Consider the case of a medical assistant who administers an allergy shot, dismisses the client, and hastens on to the next task without keeping the client under observation for 20 minutes. The client collapses in the parking lot a few minutes later as a result of anaphylactic shock from the injection. The physician-employer is responsible for the negligence of the medical assistant. The medical assistant is also liable, and both can be sued.

IN THE NEWS

Some state statutes authorize civil action if a practitioner fails to honor an advance directive or a living will. Failure to honor a client's wishes is seen as an invasion of that individual's right to consent to end-of-life decisions and deem that battery or an intentional tort has occurred. Most states provide immunity for practitioners who refuse to comply with an advance directive or living will as a matter of conscience so long as the client is referred to a practitioner who will act under the directive or living will.

▲ CRITICAL THINKING EXERCISE

A woman in her 80s, recovering from hip surgery, returns to her physician's office for a checkup. The medical assistant is cautious to make certain the woman's walker is carefully placed over the scales. With chart and pen in hand, the MA stands to the right of the client on the scales. While the medical assistant is recording the weight, the woman steps back and falls backward off the scales. Her hip is re-injured, and there are other injuries as well. The instant the medical assistant turns to enter data in the chart, the fall occurs. The client and her family are suing the physician as well as the medical assistant.

The physician is responsible for ensuring that all employees perform only those tasks within the scope of their knowledge and training. However, the employer's responsibility does not diminish employees' responsibility to perform any acts within the scope of their knowledge and training. In some cases both the physician and the employee can be found liable if injury occurs to the client as a result of the employee's actions.

The physician's employee has a responsibility to question an order if there is good reason, and a prudent employee in such a position would do so. If the order is not questioned and negligence occurs as a result, both the physician and the employee may be liable.

Professional liability is a concern of all health professionals, but physicians are most concerned because they are in a position of higher authority and responsibility.

Statute of Limitations

State legislatures have established statutes of limitations that restrict the time allowed for individuals to initiate any type of legal action. The length of time allowed for starting a lawsuit varies greatly from state to state, generally ranging from 1 to 6 years depending on the severity of the offense.

The statute of limitations most commonly begins at the time when the negligent act was allegedly committed; when the patient discovered or should have discovered the alleged negligence; or when the care, treatment, or client–physician relationship ended. However, states have differing statutes of limitations. Health care professionals should understand their state's law on the subject, as well as how the law has been interpreted in case law. Tort actions and contracts usually have separate statutes of limitations. The statute of limitations is typically longer for contracts than for torts.

Circumstances that may alter the statute of limitations occur with a person who is legally insane or when an individual has not yet reached the age of maturity. Therefore, a person declared legally insane will not come under the statute of limitations until the period of insanity has ended. In the case of minors, the period in the statute may not apply until the child has reached the age of maturity, usually 18. This fact is of special concern to pediatricians and obstetricians.

Physicians and their employees must concern themselves with the statute of limitations when considering the retention of their medical records, as well as when they could be involved in a malpractice suit. Legal counsel should be sought for interpretations and advice. Refer to Web Resources at the end of the chapter for state's statute of limitations related to injuries.

Professional Liability/Malpractice Insurance

The need for physicians to carry professional liability insurance is obvious for numerous reasons. The most important, perhaps, is financial protection. Some states mandate the minimum amount of professional liability insurance that a physician must carry.

Physicians need liability insurance protection whether they are employees or employers. For example, employment in a corporation, a health maintenance organization, or a hospital does not guarantee professional liability coverage. Many employers or institutions carry professional liability insurance merely on themselves or the institution, not on their employees. Some hospitals require a minimum amount of professional liability insurance before hospital privileges are granted. In some cases, clients sue both the employer and the employee. If employees are covered by an employer's liability policy, they should be specifically named. Employees ought to carry their own professional liability insurance. For example, medical assistants who are members of the American Association of Medical Assistants may purchase professional and personal liability insurance through the organization.

As employers, physicians need professional liability insurance mainly because of the doctrine of *respondeat superior.* Physicians may not be directly negligent, but they are liable for the acts of their employees.

Another reason for carrying professional liability insurance is that the physician may be asked for medical advice or assistance from friends or neighbors in a "casual situation." For example, at an outdoor barbecue, a neighbor may ask the physician, "My back is killing me. What can I do?" In the case of strangers, medical care may be emergent, and the physician may be the only one available to provide the care. An employer's or institution's policy probably will not cover the physician in these situations. The Good Samaritan Law, which may be applied to these situations, will be discussed later.

The kind and amount of liability coverage a physician varies according to the type of practice, the community economic level, the level of risk of the specialty, and the claims-consciousness of the clients. Most professional liability policies, however, should address (1) what the insurer will pay, (2) effective policy dates, (3) the power of the insurer in obtaining legal counsel, (4) the power of the insurer in seeking settlement, (5) what costs are covered, and (6) how payment is to be made. The policy will specify monetary limits for each claim. For example, a policy may have professional medical liability of 1 million dollars for each claim and 3 million dollars aggregate as a total amount.

Some physicians are limiting their practice and their professional liability insurance coverage because of the high cost of premiums. For example, a family practitioner may choose not to perform surgeries, thus reducing the cost of professional liability insurance.

States have been diligent in writing legislation that would limit or control the monetary amounts awarded to plaintiffs in malpractice claims, but have largely been unsuccessful. Even in states that have been successful in tort reform legislation, the cost of professional liability insurance has decreased only a little. There is a report that one physician paid a premium of $23,000 in 2002, $47,000 in 2003, and $84,000 in 2004. Another report indicates that an OB/GYN in Florida could expect to pay $201,000 in premiums in 2002, but an OB/GYN in Minnesota paid only $17,000 for the same coverage. What is the difference? How long can the increase continue? Physicians say the rate hikes are not about lawsuits, but about insurance companies making up for investment losses. Insurance companies generally decline to reveal how premiums are established, but insist that skyrocketing rates are related to the increasing costs of health care and clients litigious nature to sue.

Alternatives to Litigation

Some physicians and institutions have tried solving the malpractice dilemma by **alternative dispute resolution (ADR)** methods such as arbitration and mediation. These methods eliminate the use of the court system. The client voluntarily agrees, sometimes in advance, with the physician or institution to permit a neutral person or persons to arbitrate the case. The parties involved generally select the impartial third party, who is an expert in the area of controversy. In most instances, the decision of the arbitrator is binding, and there is limited judicial review of the process. In mediation, there is no third party; rather, the mediator is selected by both parties and attempts to facilitate negotiation between them.

A number of states have statutes addressing the use of arbitration and mediation. Some states have established centers for such alternatives to litigation. Generally, the cost of arbitration and mediation is less and will save time for both parties. The case, too, may remain more private.

Risk Management

Generally, if a healthy client–physician relationship exists, malpractice suits are not likely to occur. Some helpful guidelines to prevent malpractice include the following:

Prevention Within the Ambulatory Health Care Setting
1. Perform within the scope of training and education; do not give advice.
2. Comply with all state and federal regulations and statutes, including HIPAA.
3. Keep the office safe and equipment in readiness.
4. Diligently practice universal precautions.
5. Log telephone calls. Return all calls to clients within a reasonable time.
6. Have all diagnostic test results viewed and initialed by the physician before filing.
7. Select employees carefully, and encourage a team approach.
8. Keep all matters related to client care confidential.
9. Follow up on missed or canceled appointments and documents.
10. Continue to grow professionally.
11. Formally document (a) withdrawing from a case (Fig. 5–3) and (b) discharging clients.
12. Keep accurate and meticulous records.
13. Limit practice to scope of training and to a manageable number of clients.
14. Chart when clients are called with test results.
15. Chart all canceled appointments and no-shows.
16. Always retain original records or radiographs.
17. Have physician review files before sending accounts to collection.
18. Help your physician-employer turn your reception area into an education area.
19. Continue to increase your computer literacy.
20. Document, document, document.

Prevention with Clients
1. Practice uninterrupted listening during the critical first 60 seconds of any physician–client communication.
2. Provide an opportunity for clients to ask questions.
3. Provide time- and action-specific instructions at the close of the client contact and indicate the expected time for follow-up or recovery.
4. Put verbal instructions in writing, and give a copy to the client.
5. Do not criticize other practitioners.
6. Explain any appointment delays. Do not keep clients waiting more than 20 minutes.
7. Discuss fees before treatment.
8. Treat all persons equally.
9. Never guarantee a cure.
10. Secure informed consent.
11. Listen to clients, and always tell the physician when there is a complaint.
12. Call clients at home the day after outpatient surgery to check on their progress. Document the follow-up in the client's chart.
13. Tell clients how to get care on nights and weekends.
14. Regularly survey clients for satisfaction and follow suggestions for improvement.

REMEMBER... The Bayer Institute for Health Care recommends the 4 Es of client interaction. They are: (1) engage, (2) empathize, (3) educate, and (4) enlist clients in management of their health care. These suggestions can further help in risk management.

▲ CRITICAL THINKING EXERCISE

As office manager, you want to find ways to improve your clients' satisfaction in your large clinic. You know of a company that 'infiltrates' your clinic and actually 'pretends' to be some of your clients. The company's 'clients' call to make appointments, come in to see your physicians, use your laboratories, and other ancillary services. A report is made to the employers. It becomes an on-going practice to help you identify areas for improvement. You use the report to educate your staff. If you are a staff person, what do you think of this? Should the results be used in the employee evaluations?

Summary

Much additional information could be added to the topics in this chapter. The data included should be sufficient to assist physicians and health care employees to understand basic litigation. If office litigation becomes a reality, however, seek professional legal advice promptly.

Employees ought to maintain a **tickler file** of all important dates to recall. These include due dates for license renewals, insurance premiums, and narcotics registrations. Established patterns must be maintained for drug inventory and accurate records. Detailed descriptions and examples of such activities in the office's procedure manual are most helpful.

QUESTIONS FOR REVIEW

1. Name the requirements physicians must meet to obtain a license.

_____

_____

_____

2. Describe standard of care.

_____

_____

_____

3. Identify the meaning of confidentiality as it relates to HIPAA.

_____

_____

_____

4. List the elements that need to be included in a client–physician contract.

_____

_____

_____

5. Give an example of abandonment.

_____

_____

_____

6. Compare and contrast tort, intentional tort, and professional negligence.

_____

_____

_____

7. Name the four Ds of negligence.

_____

_____

_____

8. Give an example of when _respondeat superior_ can be used in a civil case.

_____

_____

_____

9. Define injury-related statute of limitations.

_____

_____

_____

10. What might physicians expect to pay for professional liability insurance?

_____

_____

_____

11. A physician's employee carries professional liability insurance for what reason?

_____

_____

_____

CLASSROOM EXERCISES

1. For each area of liability discussed in this chapter, give an example that might occur in ambulatory health care.

2. Ben LaPaglia, your physician's client, who is a practicing attorney, is being weighed on the scale in the hallway. He looks up and sees the daily client's schedule posted by the physician's office door. He says to you, "Is that where you always post the schedule?" Discuss.

3. Research tort reform in your state. Describe your findings.

4. When interviewing for a medical office position that bears much responsibility, you learn that the office professional liability insurance does not cover employees. What options are open to you?

5. Generally, one of three situations will determine when the injury-related statute of limitations begins. Identify them.

6. What might constitute license revocation?

7. In the vignette "Who Has a Right To Know?" could the program coordinator do anything more than speak with Nancy about her breach of confidentiality? Discuss.

REFERENCES

1. Washington Physician's Guide to Health Law, Washington State Medical Association, in association with Mary H. Spillane, Esq., Jan C. Kirkwood, Esq.; Seattle, WA, March 2001.
2. High Cost of Malpractice Insurance. Leesburg, VA, April 2, 2004. www.cbsnews.com
3. United States General Accounting Office, Report to Congressional Requestors. Medical Malpractice: Implications of Rising Premiums on Access to Health Care. August 2003. www.gao.gov

WEB RESOURCES

▲ Statute of Limitations by State. www.edgarsny.com/resources/statute-limitations
▲ The instant access to the minds of medicine. Emedicine www.emedicine.com

CHAPTER 6

Public Duties

" *The return from your work must be the satisfaction which that work brings with you and the world's need of that work. With this, life is heaven, or as near heaven as you can get. Without this—with work which you despise, which bores you, and which the world does not need—this life is hell.* "

William Edward Burghardt Du Bois

KEY TERMS

autopsy Examination by specially trained medical personnel of the body after death to determine cause of death or pathologic conditions.

coroner An official, usually elected, who investigates death from sudden, unknown, or violent causes; may or may not be a physician.

fiduciary A trustee relationship between individuals.

intimate partner violence (IPV) Intimate partner violence refers to violence/abuse between a spouse or former spouse; boyfriend, girlfriend, or former boyfriend/girlfriend; same-sex or heterosexual intimate partner, or former same-sex or heterosexual intimate partner.

notifiable or reportable disease A disease that concerns the public welfare and requires reporting to the proper authority; a potentially pathologic condition that may be transmitted directly or indirectly from one individual to another.

notifiable or reportable injury An injury that concerns the public welfare and requires reporting to the proper authority; for example, injuries resulting from gun or knife wounds.

Upon successful completion of this chapter, you will be able to:

1. Define key terms.
2. List at least five areas of public duties for physicians.
3. Discuss, in your own words, the importance of completing birth and death certificates.
4. Identify three circumstances in which a county coroner or medical examiner would be called to investigate a death.
5. Discuss the importance of prompt reporting of the death of a client.
6. Describe the process necessary for reporting communicable and notifiable diseases.
7. Restate the protocol to use for reporting adverse events to vaccines and toxoids.
8. List at least four injuries that are reportable.
9. Discuss child and elder abuse laws.
10. Identify four types of professionals who are required to report suspected child abuse.
11. Summarize intimate partner violence.
12. Describe the process used in gathering and securing evidence in the health care setting.
13. Explain, in your own words, the problem of substance abuse.
14. List four possible ways to prevent substance abuse in health care.
15. Discuss Good Samaritan Laws.

Vignette: Does the Good Samaritan law apply?

A patient underwent elective surgery for total hip replacement. Early during the surgery, the assistant surgeon became so ill he had to lie down on the operating room floor. The hospital called another physician (Dr. Howard), who had his office across the street from the hospital. He canceled his office appointments, came to the hospital, and completed the surgery with the surgeon. After the surgery, the patient suffered complications and sued Dr. Howard.

OUTCOME: Under the Good Samaritan law in California, the court ruled that Dr. Howard "did not commit any willful act or omission" while assisting the surgeon. Dr. Howard was rendering emergency care in "good faith," which addresses the quality of the intentions and not the quality of the care delivered. Also, Dr. Howard had no preexisting duty of professional care to this patient; the patient was not an established patient of his. This is another requirement of the Good Samaritan law. Further, the court stated that, as a matter of public policy, the Good Samaritan law encourages physicians to respond to emergency requests. *PERKINS V HOWARD,* 283 CAL RPTR 764 (1991).

NOTE: Although this case involves physicians working in a hospital, the legal implications are strong for ambulatory care professionals as well.

Physicians, as licensed professionals, must follow certain statutory and regulatory requirements. Reports of births; stillbirths; deaths; communicable diseases; specific injuries; and child, intimate partner, elder, and substance abuse are a few examples. Reporting requirements vary among states. Health care employees must be familiar with these statutes and regulations. To become familiar with your particular state's reporting requirements, refer to the state's statutes and administrative regulations, which are available via the Internet. Reference librarians can offer valuable help in locating the appropriate statute. In addition, health care employees may be able to contact the local and state medical associations. Most medical associations have an attorney "on call" who can offer practical guidance. Your own professional organization may offer legal assistance as well. Contact your local and state health departments and local law enforcement for reporting forms and information. Each agency may be willing to provide information.

Good Samaritan laws are discussed in this chapter so that physicians and their staff members realize that their professional responsibility goes beyond the health care setting.

Gathering and reporting statistical data and information may become an impersonal task, but physicians and their staff need to remember that these data represent individuals. Therefore the task is a personal matter. Deaths, rapes, and abuse are sensitive issues. Individuals involved need special care.

▲ CRITICAL THINKING EXERCISE

Consider your responsibilities if the following circumstances were to occur in your clinic:

1. A young husband, grieving his wife's sudden death, is told that the cause of death is still undetermined pending laboratory results.
2. A 68-year-old widow is seen today by your physician after a sexual assault.
3. The owner of a local restaurant has just tested positive for infectious hepatitis. He cannot return to work during the infectious period.

Establish policies regarding public duties including the inquiry and reporting process. Each employee should know what kind of inquiry to make, how reporting is done, who is responsible, what information is required, and when and where the report is filed. A copy should always be kept for the facility. Be knowledgeable of any community agencies that are available to provide information for the clinic and to provide valuable services for the clients.

Births and Deaths

The recording of births and deaths is an important function of the physician or provider. These certificates are legal documents and require truthfulness and prompt and proper completion. In some states, a criminal penalty will result if birth or death certificates are not properly completed. Some states refuse to accept certificates completed in inks other than black; others refuse to accept a certificate with any blanks.

A birth certificate will be used throughout a person's life to prove age, parentage, and citizenship. For example, a child will need a birth certificate when entering school. Adults will require a birth certificate to register to vote or to obtain a driver's license, a marriage license, a passport, veteran's benefits, welfare aid, and Social Security benefits.

Certificate requirements vary from state to state. A stillbirth or fetal death, in which the fetus has not reached the 20th week of gestation, may require neither a birth nor a death certificate. In some states, however, a special stillbirth form is used; in others, it is necessary to file both a birth and death certificate. If the birth is considered a live birth and then the infant dies, both a standard birth and death certificate need to be completed.

In the event of a non-hospital birth, the person in attendance is responsible for initiating the birth certificate. In such a delivery, a parent should verify that the process is completed according to state regulations.

Check with your state's health or vital statistics department, which offers information regarding reporting of birth and death certificates. This agency provides detailed information for completing the standard forms.

Generally speaking, physicians sign a certificate giving the cause of death of the deceased upon whom they have been in professional attendance. Otherwise, someone of greater authority, such as the county health officer or **coroner** will assume the responsibility. In some states, a physician is forbidden by law to sign certain death certificates. Examples include, but are not limited to, a death caused by criminal activity, a death without a physician present, a death from an undetermined cause, or a violent or unlawful death. These cases are immediately turned over to a coroner, medical examiner, or equivalent official for investigation and issuance of a death certificate. A death may also need to be reported to the coroner in the following instances: a death occurring within 24 hours after a client is admitted to a hospital or licensed health care facility, nonattendance by a physician during the 3 days before death, or death of an individual outside a hospital or licensed health care facility. The physician should not send the remains to a mortician without authorization from the next of kin or other person responsible for funeral expenses.

Prompt reporting by the physician is required so that the remains will not be disturbed and evidence will not be lost. This is particularly significant if an investigation or **autopsy** is to be performed. The physician may be the only one who knows the client's current medical history and treatment. As such, when called to the death scene, the physician may discover facts inconsistent with the client's medical history and can then notify the authorities. Law enforcement may begin an investigation resulting in prosecution of criminals and alteration of survivors' rights or other benefits. Also, if the death is the result of an accident or an occupational or environmental hazard, an autopsy or investigation may identify the actual cause of death. Thus the physician is a key individual in the discovery of facts surrounding death, and prompt reporting is essential.

As a courtesy to the family, it is imperative that the death certificate be completed and signed as quickly as possible so that funeral and financial arrangements can begin. Many states have a requirement that the death certificate be filed within 24 to 72 hours. The physician's office staff should realize that no arrangements can be made until the death certificate is signed.

The death certificate proves a person has died. A certified copy of a death certificate is generally necessary in obtaining access to insurance policy monies, bank accounts, safe-deposit boxes, dispersal of estates, real estate transactions, tax base information, Internal Revenue Service information, Social Security and veteran's benefits.

Communicable and Notifiable Diseases

A disease is reportable (**notifiable or reportable disease**) when it concerns the public welfare and when it is a potentially pathologic condition that may be transmitted directly or indirectly from one individual to another. The reporting of communicable diseases varies among states; however, local health departments publish and periodically update lists of 30 or more notifiable diseases and the required reporting format.

Physicians have the duty to report notifiable diseases by phone, by mail, or electronically. Reports are usually made by the office assistant, who telephones the local health department and furnishes the following information:

1. Disease (or suspected disease)
2. Name, address, age, and occupation of person with suspected disease
3. Date of onset of disease
4. Name of person reporting

To report by mail, use the appropriate case report cards furnished by the health department. Many diseases are reported on special forms. A check with your local health department may reveal 20 or more specific forms for diseases. Some states encourage reporting by phone, with the statistical data being collected by the health department. Other states require that the initial paperwork be completed at the time the notifiable disease is detected. Whatever method of reporting is used, be prompt, consistent, factual, and complete. Keep a copy of the report for the files. The health department will attempt to determine the source of infection and mode of transmission so that public health will be protected. The list in Box 6.1 is not exhaustive; however, it identifies those communicable diseases that most threatens public safety.

▲ B O X 6.1 **Communicable and Infectious Diseases Commonly Reported Immediately by Telephone**

Any case of an unusual illness thought to have public health implications

Anthrax	Plague
Botulism	Poliomyelitis
Cholera	Rabies
Diphtheria	Rubeola
Encephalitis	Tetanus
Hepatitis A	Typhoid
Pertussis	Typhus

Childhood and Adolescent Vaccinations

All health care providers who administer certain childhood vaccines and toxoids are required by law to record certain information and report adverse events. In 1986, Congress passed the National Childhood Vaccine Injury Act identifying vaccines and toxoids that require specific documentation. The information to be recorded includes the date of the vaccine's administration; the manufacturer and lot number of the vaccine; and the name, address, and title of the person administering the vaccine. Any adverse events after administration would also be recorded. Pediatric offices offer written information to parents and guardians about vaccines and toxoids and many require signed informed consent forms before administration of vaccines.

▲ CRITICAL THINKING EXERCISE

Discuss the premise that global/world vaccinations help to stop the spread of disease into industrialized nations. Are any difficulties associated with global/world vaccinations? With vaccinations in the United States? Explain.

BOX 6.2 **Recommended Childhood Immunizations**

According to the American Academy of Pediatrics and the American Academy of Family Physicians, the recommended childhood immunizations as of 2006 are as follows:

Diphtheria, tetanus, and pertussis
Measles, mumps, and rubella
Poliovirus inactivated
Hepatitis A
Hepatitis B
H. influenzae type b
Influenza
Meningococcal
Pneumococcal
Varicella

For more detailed information, consult your health department or the Internet. This list is not exhaustive, however, it identifies those communicable diseases that most threaten public safety.

Notifiable or Reportable Injury

An injury is reportable (**notifiable or reportable injury**) when it concerns the public welfare and requires reporting to the proper authority; for example, injuries resulting from gun or knife wounds. Some states have detailed requirements for reporting injuries. Others have none. Check with the local and state medical associations and law enforcement agencies for specific information.

Generally, however, injuries caused by lethal weapons, such as guns and knives, are always reported and persons are usually treated in emergency or hospital facilities. When persons who have been raped or battered, seek and receive treatment from ambulatory health care physicians, they may be referred immediately to the emergency room of a local hospital.

Questions may arise concerning reporting requirements. For example, if an adult rape survivor reports for medical care in an ambulatory health care facility after an assault, must the assault be reported? If the physician suspects abuse, must it be reported? At least 50 state variances govern the reporting of such incidents. In some states, marital rape laws may mandate reporting of spousal abuse. In these states, failure to report child, elder, and spousal abuse may specifically be considered a misdemeanor. Information that follows is important for the health professional in identifying and recognizing abuse and violence.

Abuse

The responsibilities and tasks performed in the health care setting can sometimes be very stressful. Abuse is one of the most serious of those stressors. Emotions are especially charged when there is evidence of child or elder abuse, but are equally as difficult to hold in check when there is abuse in family or close personal relationships. The most difficult task may not be in treating the individual abused, but in remaining calm and nonjudgmental about the circumstances that bring the abused and/or the abuser to the health care setting.

Child Abuse

 Culturally the issue is complex because there is the belief in a majority of cultures that parents are best able to provide for the care and discipline of their children. There may be the belief that parents have a moral obligation to correct a child's misbehavior. The idea of "spare the rod, spoil the child" is a paraphrase from a Bible scripture. The Mother Goose rhymes some learned as children express the frustration of the old woman in a shoe who did not know what to do with all her children, so she "whipped them all soundly and put them to bed." Incidents of child abuse and neglect may be seen in a hospital or a physician's or provider's office when a child displays fractures, burns, severe bruises, and questionable injuries. Not so obvious injuries may include dislocations, cerebrospinal trauma, and internal injuries resulting from blows to the abdomen. Malnutrition, lower than expected growth rate, poor hygiene, gross dental problems, and unattended medical needs also may indicate neglect or abuse.

Definitions of child abuse are essential for understanding what is to be reported.

Neglect: Failure to provide for basic care including food, clothing, shelter, or medical attention that endangers the health of the child.

Physical Injury: Burns, severe bruising, lacerations, fractures, injuries to internal organs, serious bodily injury. Injury is often obvious.

Mental Injury: Harm to a child's well-being that damages their psychological or intellectual development. Child may be emotionally withdrawn, depressed, anxious, or aggressive, but injury is not obvious.

Sexual Abuse: Using a child to engage in sexual activity of any sort to include rape, molestation, incest, prostitution, or sexual exploitation. Physical evidence may be present.

Sexually Explicit Conduct: Actual or simulated sexual intercourse with a child (same sex or opposite sex), masturbation, exhibition of genitalia, or sadistic or masochistic abuse. Likely is not obvious to health care professionals.

Child Molestation: Oral-genital contact, viewing and fondling of genitals. Likely is not obvious to health care professionals.

Sexual Exploitation: Child pornography, child prostitution, sexual explicit use of child's image in electronic media. Likely is not obvious to health care professionals.

Incest: Sexual relations between children or parents in the same family. May be recognized by health care professionals.

All 50 states and the District of Columbia have laws that mandate the reporting of child abuse and neglect. The report is made to an agency named in the state statute. Certain individuals are required to report suspected abuse and neglect. These include health professionals, social service personnel, law enforcement personnel, educators, and any professional person working with children. Some states also allow a hospital administrator or a physician to detain a child legally without a guardian's consent in such instances. Individuals making the report are protected from civil and criminal liability if the report is found to be false. Failure to report is a misdemeanor in some states. The function of reporting is to identify incidents of suspected abuse and neglect, not to prove abuse or neglect. The report may be oral, written, or both. Immediate reporting is paramount so that a proper investigation can be initiated. Information required in the report may include the following:

1. Name, address, and age of child
2. Name and address of child's parents (or guardians)
3. Nature and extent of the injury, neglect, or abuse

4. Any evidence of previous incidents of abuse or neglect, including their nature and extent
5. Any other information that may be helpful in establishing the cause of the child's injuries, neglect, or death and the identity of the perpetrator(s)

If a crime has been committed, law enforcement must be notified.

IN THE NEWS

The Human Rights Watch organization states that governments around the world are breaking promises to children. For examples, they cite, among others, the following:

1. A very large number of children are used for commercial sexual purposes every year, often ending up with HIV/AIDS or other sexually transmitted diseases. Prostituted children can be raped, beaten, sodomized, emotionally abused, tortured, and even killed by pimps.
2. Street children are subjected to routine harassment and physical abuse by police, government, and private security forces. The children face extortion, theft, severe beatings, mutilation, sexual abuse, and even death.

Intimate Partner Violence

For many years, the terms spousal abuse and domestic violence have been used. Today **intimate partner violence (IPV)** more accurately describes the problem. Intimate partner violence refers to violence/abuse between a spouse or former spouse; boyfriend, girlfriend, or former boyfriend/girlfriend; same-sex or heterosexual intimate partner, or former same-sex or heterosexual intimate partner. IPV refers to actual or threatened physical, sexual, or psychological harm to another individual. The term "survivor" rather than "victim" is used because survivor is believed to be a more appropriate and empowering term.

 Four main types of IPV are identified:

1. Physical violence is the intent to do harm, cause disability, injury, or death. Some examples include hitting, pushing, grabbing, biting, punching, slapping, restraining, burning, or using a weapon and one's strength to hurt another person.
2. Sexual violence is forcing another to commit a sex act against his or her will; having sex with someone who is unable to understand, decline participation, or say "no" because he/she is disabled or under the influence of alcohol or drugs; having abusive sexual contact.
3. Threats of physical or sexual violence occur when gestures, words, or weapons are used to cause harm, injury, disability, or death.
4. Psychological/emotional violence refers to trauma that includes humiliation, control, any acts to embarrass or diminish a partner, isolating a partner from family and friends, and denying access to monetary funds or basic resources.

Another form of IPV has been added called *stalking*. Stalking is the act of following, spying upon, making repeated calls or contacts after being asked not to, appearing at one's home or place of employment, and making threats, with or without a weapon.

No one knows for certain how much IPV occurs because not all incidences are reported. Men as well as women may be abusers; however, more women than men are abused. IPV is a criminal offense in some states. Not all states require IPV to be reported; often it depends upon whether a weapon is used. Any form of IPV that is acknowledged in the care setting will have to be reported when required to do so. All attempts should be made to keep the survivor as safe as possible. Referral and resources should be made available to survivors who seek protection.

Rape

Rape, a crime of violence, is forced sexual intercourse or penetration of a bodily orifice by a penis or some other object. If a weapon is used, aggravated criminal assault has occurred. One or more persons may commit rape against an individual, and gang rape can involve several individuals. Rape is a reportable criminal act.

 Rape creates a serious crisis for survivors who are likely to react to the experience in four phases.

1. *Disorganization* phase of fear, shock, denial, and a feeling of loss of control.
2. *Denial* phase when the survivor outwardly appears normal, but inwardly has suppressed the incident; gradually begins to gain control.
3. *Reorganization* phase is when the survivor is no longer in denial, but often becomes depressed; may feel a need to talk about the rape.
4. *Recovery* phase is when survivors realize they are not to blame for the rape.

It helps if survivors are able to vent their feelings of anger, guilt, and shame during the recovery process. Women and girls are more often raped than men. Men and boys, however, are more likely to be gang raped.

Elder Abuse

Intentional or unintentional harm, physically or psychologically, of someone 60 years of age or older is termed elder abuse. The elderly may be more vulnerable than others because of their social isolation and mental impairment. Their abusers may include professional caregivers, family members, partners, doctors, lawyers, bankers, accountants, or strangers. Elder abuse may occur anywhere, but is more commonly found in the home, a nursing home, or other institution.

 The types of elder abuse are as follows:

Neglect: Careless lack of attention that results in harm. Neglect may be emotional or physical. Examples include withholding medication or necessary medical attention, personal care, food and water, or any basic necessities of life. Abandonment, lack of assistance with mobility, failure to provide adequate diaper changes, and insufficient help with hygiene or bathing constitutes neglect.

Physical Abuse: Violence that results in bodily harm or severe mental stress. Assault, beating, whipping, hitting, punching, pushing, shoving, pinching, force-feeding, shaking, rough handling during caregiving are some of the examples of physical abuse.

Financial Abuse: Financial or material exploitation of an elder's resources. The improper use of money, assets, or property is financial abuse. Examples include withdrawing cash from accounts without permission, cashing checks received (e.g., pension and Social Security) and denying those funds to the elder, forcing an elder to alter a will, and forging a senior's signature.

Emotional/Psychological Abuse: Actions that dehumanize an elderly person including social isolation, name-calling, harassment, humiliating, insulting, threatening to punish, treating an elderly person like a child, and yelling or screaming. This form of abuse usually accompanies one of the other forms.

Sexual Abuse: Any sexual contact with an elder without his or her permission, including fondling, touching, kissing, forcing the elder to observe sexual acts, rape or sodomy, spying on the elder in the bathroom or bedroom, and coerced nudity.

IN THE NEWS

Dr. Terry Hill, medical director of a San Francisco hospital and clinical professor, states that elder mistreatment feeds the liability crises. In 1998 a California law passed mandating that physicians report incidents that reasonably appear to involve abuse or neglect. Lawsuits followed. In one lawsuit, twelve nursing home employees were arrested on felony charges of elder abuse during a sting operation involving video cameras. Some California physicians are concerned that they would face charges for not reporting and some are turning away from elder care because they are frustrated by the lawsuits, the struggles for malpractice coverage, and the environment of suspicion. What legal and ethical concerns does this raise?

The majority of states have enacted legislation addressing elder abuse or abuse of vulnerable adults. The laws generally name a health care professional as one who reports the abuse, and in some states, it is a requirement to report the suspected abuse. States may protect the reporter of suspected elder abuse from civil and criminal liability. The reporting agency varies in each state but generally is a social or welfare agency, a long-term-care facility or police or ombudsperson. Risk factors for elder abuse include advanced age, female gender, and dependence on a caregiver, social isolation, behavior problems, and increased physical and mental impairment.

REMEMBER... Basic considerations when dealing with the assault survivor include the following:

1. Consider the vulnerability to future assault. Physicians may feel an ethical obligation and choose to intervene. Such intervention might include questioning the possibility of abuse, discussing safety options, providing a list of community referrals and resources, giving therapeutic support, and documenting the situation for future reference.
2. Respect the survivor's right not to report abuse if this is permissible by law.
3. Remember that both the survivor and the abuser need professional care and have rights protected by law.

Caring for individuals who have been abused is emotionally difficult; requirements for reporting abuse will vary by state. Urban areas have community service agencies such as rape relief and sexual assault centers. The physician may refer the survivor to such an agency for additional, specialized services. However, if these services are unavailable or the survivor chooses to be treated by the physician alone, the physician needs information from law enforcement agencies regarding reporting the incident and obtaining, securing, and handling medicolegal evidence.

The survivor should be treated as soon as possible after the injury or assault, not only for the survivor's welfare but also to preserve evidence of possible criminal acts. Rape survivors need to feel supported and cared for and to feel that the violent act will make no difference in how they are treated by people.

▲ CRITICAL THINKING EXERCISE

 Identify cultures in which abuse (child, intimate partner, adult, elder, substance) is defined differently. For example, consider the following:

1. The use of a belt to spank a child
2. A cultural attitude that recommends circumcision of young girls (removal of clitoris and suturing of the vaginal opening)
3. A culture in which the use of illegal drugs may result in beheading

4. A culture that severely punishes a rapist and financially and emotionally supports the female survivor or a child born of that rape
5. A culture that kills its infants if they are infirm and there is not enough food and shelter available

Evidence

Gathering of evidence is more likely to occur in the emergency room or hospital setting. Situations will arise in the ambulatory health care setting, however, in which employees and physicians need to be knowledgeable about the methods of proper collection and preservation of evidence. (See Chapter 4 for an explanation of the trial process.) When in doubt, seek professional guidance from attorneys and the proper authorities.

In the ambulatory health care setting, physicians may gather legal evidence knowingly or unknowingly. Later they may be asked to offer the evidence or may be subpoenaed to give the evidence. Office situations in which evidence will be collected include the female child's urinalysis showing sperm, the young boy when he is receiving medical treatment reveals he has been gang raped, or a client entering with a superficial knife wound. The circumstances just described may involve physicians as witnesses in litigation; therefore, proper examination and documentation are essential.

One of the first ways evidence is documented is through medical records. Malpractice lawsuits are commonly lost because of improper documentation in medical records. Specifically, providers must record the time of client arrival; a complete explanation of the client's condition, both physical and emotional; and what was done for the client. Obviously, treatment and care of the client is primary, but documentation in the client's medical record must follow. The written documentation must be clear, concise, complete, and in order.

Evidence may be in the form of a complete written description, x-rays, photographs, clothing, samples for laboratory testing, or samples of foreign objects. Photographs and x-rays need to be dated and labeled with the client's name. Photographs may need a brief description relating what is pictured. Both x-rays and photographs should be stored in envelopes to protect them. Any objects and clothing must be properly and carefully removed, labeled, and stored. Clothing should not be cut unless necessary and then along seams. Do not rinse or wash clothing. In fact, wear gloves and do not handle clothing any more than necessary to avoid changing or damaging evidence. Any body fluids, such as vomitus or gastric washing, should be saved, especially in poisoning cases, for future analysis.

You may be requested by law enforcement to take client samples such as blood; semen; vaginal, oral, or rectal smears; or skin, fingernail, or hair clippings. Samples must be properly labeled and preserved. Every piece of evidence needs to be preserved as much as possible and securely stored in a locked place to avoid tampering or loss.

Having only one employee handle all evidence can prevent it from becoming inadmissible because it cannot be properly traced or verified. When giving evidence to the proper authorities, ask for a receipt for your files. Know to whom you are giving the evidence.

Physicians should cooperate with law enforcement authorities who need to talk to the client. The physician and office staff should not be overprotective of the client, nor should the client be jeopardized. The authorities need to receive information on the client so that they can begin their investigation immediately.

If a client dies in the ambulatory care facility or arrives dead, the medical examiner or coroner should be called immediately and the remains should not be touched or removed. Health care employees should not touch, tamper, or remove any tubes or paraphernalia from the client. Leave the deceased as is; otherwise, evidence may be useless to authorities.

Substance Abuse

Substance misuse or abuse is found in every sector of society. No one is exempt. It is commonplace in schools, in colleges, in all the professions, and in industry. Physicians are pestered by abusers seeking controlled substances for their personal use or for resale in the streets. Pharmacists receive fake prescription requests on the telephone, and because of that, are careful to properly identify the person calling in the prescription.

Health professionals also are vulnerable to drug and alcohol abuse, perhaps more so to drugs because of their availability in the workplace. However, physicians and their employees have a public duty to be alert to substance abuse and to do everything possible to prevent its increase.

The abuse of alcohol may be detected in the health care setting when clients are asked about their drinking habits. Whether the drug of choice is alcohol, prescription medications, or illicit street drugs, the approach is the same. Substance abuse of any kind is injurious to the health and well-being of clients. Health care professionals who have the most success with such clients will be the ones who are able to honestly discuss the abuse issues and possible treatment plans without judgment or condemnation.

A common problem in the health care setting is a drug abuser securing the same prescription drug from more than one physician and pharmacy in an area. Often abusers go from door to door at medical clinics with a convincing tale of woe or a set of symptoms that may warrant a prescription drug. The abuser may convince the office assistant that this is a valid complaint and the assistant is then coerced into becoming an advocate for the abuser. Another problem occurs when a physician becomes what is known as a "script doctor," one who freely and excessively prescribes potentially dangerous drugs.

Some communities have established hot lines so that descriptions of suspected drug abusers and their mode of operation can be communicated to legal authorities. However, be aware of HIPAA regulations and client confidentiality. One technique that works well is for the assistant or physician to ask for picture identification from each new client. Most abusers will not produce such identification. An assistant should also be advised that the physician will authorize no controlled substance prescriptions without first seeing the client.

Physicians and office staff must keep prescription pads secure. Controlled substances should not be kept on the premises unless necessary. Any that are kept must be locked and immediately reported if stolen or lost. Be alert to the regular client who may be seeing more than one doctor for the same complaint and receiving several prescriptions. Carefully question clients during examination.

The market for prescription drugs on the street is a lucrative one. The abuse of prescription medications, especially by young adults, is rampant. Teens steal their parents' medicine, take them to school, and sell them for more potent and illicit drugs, or take the medications themselves. Young adults have learned that street drugs may be laced with very dangerous and poisonous substances and are very costly, while stolen prescriptive medications are considered free and safe.

A frank, honest discussion must be conducted with young adults that encourages saying "no" to alcohol and drugs; yet, health care professionals must be careful to keep an open dialog so that their clients are comfortable in admitting any substance abuse problems. This kind of discussion is best held when parents or guardians are not present.

Physicians and health professionals must establish firm and clear procedures to curb the increase of substance abuse. A comprehensive substance abuse history should be taken from all clients. Clients may come with a current substance abuse condition in addition to another disease or illness so both must be addressed. It is imperative for health care professionals to be knowledgeable of signs and symptoms of substance abuse and report them to the physician. If it is the health care professional that abuses substances, their ability to function safely will be impaired.

Refer to Chapter 8 for specific information when releasing information in medical records regarding substance abuse.

Good Samaritan Laws

Good Samaritan statutes exist in all 50 states, yet their content varies widely with regard to who is protected, the standard of care required, and the circumstances under which protection is provided. The statute itself is a legal doctrine meant to encourage physicians and health care professionals to render emergency first-aid treatment to accident victims without liability for negligence. In some states it does not apply to an emergency arising in a clinic, hospital, or office where the client–physician relationship exists. However, the scene of an emergency may include the emergency room of the hospital in the event of a medical disaster. Most Good Samaritan laws state that the person administering the aid cannot benefit financially or receive any rewards.

The Good Samaritan statutes mainly apply to physicians, but many also address other health care professionals. A few statutes include laypersons. In most states, no one, including physicians and health care professionals, has the legal obligation to render first aid in a life-threatening situation.

Most Good Samaritan statutes merely attempt to protect the physician or health care professional who gives first aid and acts "in good faith" and "without gross negligence." In some states, you must be a Good Samaritan or face a penalty; whereas in others, legislation states that physicians must administer emergency treatment to the best of their ability. In most states a professional should not leave an individual during an emergency (1) unless it is to call for assistance, or (2) until an equally competent professional is available, or (3) unless it is unsafe to continue.

The majority of Good Samaritan statutes are poorly written and leave many unanswered questions. Not many define the following: What is an emergency? What is care rendered gratuitously? Where and to what extent can care be given and be covered by the statute?

Many health care professionals are reluctant to render aid in an emergency. Reasons for this attitude may include the laws that are vague, the legal and professional advice to be cautious, and the fear that the situation may require skills outside of one's training and education. The health professional may be as anxious to avoid getting involved as the layperson. The risk of liability, however, has been grossly exaggerated. Lawsuits are rarely filed against a Good Samaritan, whether physician or health professional.

All health care professionals and their employees ought to know their Good Samaritan laws and specifically what and who they address. Certainly, the legal and ethical ramifications of rendering aid in an emergency should be considered before an emergency presents itself. Although the health care professional may feel inadequate and unprotected in an emergency, the general public considers such a professional to be far more qualified than any layperson appearing on the scene.

Health care professionals who do render aid in an emergency must remember to treat within the scope of their training and to give adequate care in light of the circumstances. They also should take comfort in the fact that the chance of a lawsuit is slim.

REMEMBER... To protect yourself from possible liability for performing under the Good Samaritan law always act on behalf of the victim. Continue to update CPR and first aid classes. Follow your scope of practice and use common sense. Do not do anything you are not trained or educated to do. Under no circumstances accept gifts or rewards.

Summary

The health care climate of today indicates that hospitals are often full, and emergency rooms are overcrowded and understaffed. The result is that many clients turn toward their primary care provider in the ambulatory health care setting for treatment that might otherwise be seen in the hospital or emergency room. Many births take place in the home or birthing center, placing emphasis upon the attending physician or midwife to file the information for the birth certificate. Clients with communicable and reportable diseases are likely first seen in ambulatory care. Increasingly, some individuals who are abused or harmed in an abusive situation are less comfortable in the hospital emergency environment than they are with their personal primary care provider. Health care professionals must be prepared and have the appropriate knowledge and education to provide the best medical care. They must function within legal and ethical guidelines.

QUESTIONS FOR REVIEW

1. List the reasons for filing both a birth and a death certificate.

2. Restate the information required when reporting a communicable disease.

3. List the currently recommended childhood and adolescent immunizations.

4. Explain three guidelines to remember when caring for an abused client.

5. Identify the various forms of child abuse.

6. Define IPV.

_____

_____

_____

7. Compare and contrast the varying forms of elder abuse.

_____

_____

_____

8. State how you would preserve x-rays and photographs for evidence.

_____

_____

_____

9. Good Samaritan laws address what guidelines?

_____

_____

_____

10. Health care professionals who suspect substance abuse in a client need to take what kind of actions?

_____

_____

_____

CLASSROOM EXERCISES

1. Using the three examples described in the Critical Thinking Exercise at the beginning of the chapter (p. 84), discuss your responsibilities in each situation, the possible referral agencies available, and the possible problems encountered. How can you be of assistance to your physician employer?

2. What problems occur when a death certificate remains unsigned?

3. What are the future implications if a birth is not reported?

4. Explore agencies in your community for the referral of abused persons, and share your findings.

5. The physician gives you an envelope of x-rays and a sealed bag of clothing items and asks you to keep them safe until law enforcement officials arrive. How would you keep them safe? Why is this important?

6. You suspect a colleague in your clinic abuses alcohol; her early morning breath smells of alcohol, she is continually late, and her work is becoming unreliable. What action do you take?

7. Under what circumstances might a physician decide not to render emergency aid?

8. Intimate partner violence is a relatively new term. Discuss its relevance with a close friend.

9. Identify advantages and disadvantages of using the term survivor rather than victim. Which would you use? Justify your response.

WEB RESOURCES

▲ American Academy of Pediatrics: American Academy of Family Physicians; and Communicable Disease Center. Childhood Immunization Schedule and Catch-up Schedule, 2006. www.cispimmunize

▲ Communicable Disease Center. www.cdc.gov "Adult Immunization Schedule, 2005."

▲ Communicable Disease Center. www.cdc.gov "Nationally Notifiable Infectious Diseases, 2006."

▲ Medical Encyclopedia: Reportable Diseases. www.nlm.hih.gov/medlineplus

▲ Mental Health Issues. "Expert, Non-commercial information on mental health and lifelong wellness." www.helpguide.org

▲ National Birth Certificates/National Death Certificates. www.nationalbirthcertificates.com and www.nationaldeathcertificates.com

▲ National Center for Injury Prevention and Control. "Fact Sheet: Intimate Partner Violence: Overview." www.cdc.gov/factsheets

▲ New Opinions and CEJA Reports. www.ama-assn.org.ama/pub/category

▲ Shelter for Darkness. Website related to child abuse and domestic violence. www.shelterfordarkness.com

▲ Smith Law Firm, Susan K. Smith, Atty, Hartford & Avon, CT. "Mandatory Reporting of Child Abuse and Neglect." www.smith-lawfirm.com/mandatory_reporting.html

▲ The National Center for Victims of Crime. www.ncvc.org

▲ The Free Encyclopedia. http://en.wikipedia.org

CHAPTER 7

Consent

*Realize that you always have choices.
It's up to you.*

Leo Buscaglia

Upon successful completion of this chapter, you will be able to:

1. Define key terms.
2. Explain, in your own words, why consent is important.
3. Give an example of verbal consent, nonverbal consent, and written consent.
4. Compare informed and uninformed consent.
5. List the four elements of the doctrine of informed consent.
6. Identify the following special situations in consent: minors, spouses and domestic partners, language barriers, clinical research, and when consent is not necessary.
7. Discuss the role of the health care employee in the consent process.

Vignette: *When is enough enough?*

A client comes in for her annual gynecological examination. Her physician recommends she have a Pap smear, but she refuses. The physician stresses its importance and documents why it is important in the chart. The following year when the client returns for her annual examination, the physician again stresses why she needs the Pap smear. The client again refuses. Six months later the client is diagnosed with cervical cancer. Soon she files a lawsuit against the physician.

OUTCOME: The jury found the physician liable under the doctrine of informed consent for not stressing more that the client needed a Pap smear.

All health care employees are involved in the consent process with the clients they serve. Although the health care provider has the primary responsibility to inform the client of proposed treatment and to obtain consent for a procedure, clients commonly ask questions of health care employees. Consequently, everyone must understand all aspects of consent.

Consent is the voluntary affirmation by a client to allow touching, examination, or treatment by medically authorized personnel. Consent allows clients to determine what will be done with their bodies. Without consent, intentional touching can be considered a criminal offense. Consent is authorization given by implications of a client's behavior, a medical contract, or by law. Consent is obtained through word or action. Consent may be given orally, expressed by nonverbal behavior, or expressed in writing. Some state laws mandate that written consent is necessary for any invasive procedure. Further, some states may find health employees liable for failing to give information to clients and obtaining their consent. Health professionals also may be legally liable when offering information and for obtaining informed consent from clients. Know your state's **doctrine of informed consent** laws (Fig. 7–1). Consider the following examples:

1. A client calls complaining of a persistent, productive cough. When the receptionist makes the appointment with the physician, the client has given consent for examination, which may include throat examination and culture.
2. When a physician requires a blood test for diagnosis and the client comes to the laboratory with a rolled-up sleeve, implied consent is being given.
3. A client is scheduled for an office surgical procedure and signs an appropriate consent form. This action constitutes a medical contract between the client and the physician. Written consent has been obtained.
4. If a client who comes to the office suddenly stops breathing during the physician's examination, the physician will take immediate action to restore breathing and preserve life. Consent is implied by law in an emergency situation when a client is unable to give consent. An emergency is said to exist when the client is in immediate danger and action is necessary to save a life or prevent further damage.

Integral to consent is the client's belief that the health care professional to whom consent is given has the knowledge, skill, and ability to perform such tasks. In the examples above, the client has a right to expect that the physician has the ability to determine the need for a throat culture, perform the required surgery, and administer emergency treatment. Likewise, the client can expect the laboratory technician to know proper venipuncture technique.

Informed and Uninformed Consent

Two underlying reasons for obtaining informed consent are to ensure individual autonomy (the right to be left alone or the right to privacy) and to encourage rational decision-making. **REMEMBER…** Consent is a process, not a mere piece of paper or form to sign. The process implies a two-way communication between client and health care

Consent

By word	By action	Informed	Uninformed
• oral • written	• nonverbal behavior	• client understands • often is written	• client does not understand

FIGURE 7–1 The four forms of consent.

provider that will maximize the client's participation and ensure full knowledge of any procedure.

Ideally, consent is informed, with the client understanding all facets of the consent. Clients who are a party to consent usually are informed or have sufficient understanding of the circumstances surrounding their consent. **Uninformed consent** occurs when the client gives permission but does not understand or comprehend what has been consented to.

Because of the many occasions arising in the ambulatory health care setting that involve complicated medical procedures that are often difficult for clients to understand, informed consent is important to give the provider permission to act. To ensure that proper consent is obtained, it usually is put in writing. Specific guidelines generally are established in each state's doctrine of informed consent.

The Doctrine of Informed Consent

Informed consent is a client's right to know and understand before agreeing to a procedure. It is the physician's sole responsibility to obtain consent from the client, even if other staff assist in the process. Consent should be obtained in writing because written consent implies an intentional and deliberate decision.

 States vary in their doctrine of informed consent, laws but require that the client understand the nature of the illness and be told, in language easily understood, the following:

1. What the procedure is and how it is to be performed
2. The possible risks involved and the expected results
3. Any alternative procedures or treatments and their risks
4. Results if no treatment is given

Vignette: Focus on Clients

To further illustrate the necessary elements of informed consent, consider Phil, age 65, who has been diagnosed by the physician as having adenocarcinoma. His physician is careful to explain the nature of this particular disease to Phil and its possible progression in his body. The physician then outlines the possible forms of treatment, such as surgery, chemotherapy, or radiation, and carefully explains the risks of each, as well as possible outcomes. The physician frequently encourages a particular form of treatment even before the client asks for a recommendation. Here the physician has knowledge of Phil's particular case that may be expected to give credence to such a recommendation. However, the physician should be careful also to explain the possible risks of no treatment at all. Although the client looks to the physician for medical information and recommendations, the decision is the client's alone.

In Phil's situation (see "Focus on Client") as with most others, all health care professionals must be sensitive to the impact of such a decision. For consent to be meaningful, Phil may need time to comprehend the essential elements of the consent. This may include talking with family members, seeking a second opinion, considering financial implications, or just being alone. Staff members also need to be prepared to clarify, further explain, or direct additional questions to the physician if the client so indicates. Not until a later time will written consent be obtained and the physician is able to proceed. The written consent must reflect each of the elements previously described and should also contain the client's signature, the physician's signature, and the signature of a witness. The physician may ask Phil to explain in his own words what he believes is happening.

Problems in Consent

Consent may be difficult to obtain in the treatment of a **minor,** a person who has not reached the age of maturity. In some states, courts recognize two types of minors as being capable of informed consent. **Mature minors** are considered to possess sufficient understanding of treatment they are to receive and its consequences despite their chronological age. **Emancipated minors** have the legal capacity of an adult as indicated by age, maturity, intelligence, training, experience, economic independence, and freedom from parental control. In some states, someone who is married or in the military is an emancipated minor. Legal questions of capacity to consent related to both the mature minor and the emancipated minor are considered on a case-by-case basis because not all states recognize mature or emancipated minors.

In most states, minors are unable to give consent for medical care except as described previously or in special cases when minors are pregnant, request birth control or an abortion, have suspected sexually transmitted diseases, have possible problems with substance abuse, or are in need of psychiatric care. In all other situations, the provider or staff should attempt to reach the parent(s) or legal guardian(s) for consent.

 Legal implications to consider when treating a minor are as follows:

1. A minor has the right to confidentiality. A 16-year-old who seeks a prescription for birth control pills has the right for that information to be kept confidential.
2. A minor who may legally consent to treatment may not be financially responsible. If the 16-year-old in the first example does not pay when services are given, collecting from parents who have not given their consent may be difficult and breaches confidentiality.
3. A minor's legal guardian may have to be determined—a special problem in the case of divorce and remarriage. If the father of a child is financially responsible, but the child resides with the mother, who may properly give consent for treatment?

You must be knowledgeable regarding your own state's consent laws and have an attorney's recommendations when problems occur.

The law that governs consent is not well defined for minors, and it may be vague or even nonexistent with respect to spouses and/or domestic partners. Increased awareness of the rights of women and domestic partners has a significant impact on the legal system. More advances can be expected in the future. A spouse has the legal right to consent to and receive

---

IN THE NEWS

In July 2006, a 16-year-old boy was ordered by a Virginia juvenile court judge to report to a hospital to continue treatment for Hodgkin's disease. The boy and his parents wanted to try alternative therapies because of the chemotherapy side effects. However, the judge ruled that the parents were neglectful and must continue to share custody of their son with the Department of Social Services. In the state of Virginia, courts are allowed to override parental decisions if the child's health is endangered.

One month later, the day the case was to go to trial, the family and state officials reached an agreement that the boy will see a new oncologist while continuing with his alternative treatment in Mexico. In addition to using traditional therapies, the new oncologist also uses alternative therapies, focusing on nutrition. The family's attorney says that this is a good resolution. Now the new oncologist may treat the boy with radiation rather than the much opposed chemotherapy.

medical care and treatment without a spouse's approval. Domestic partners also may consent without the other partner's approval.

▲ CRITICAL THINKING EXERCISE

1. A 17-year-old ward of the court is pregnant and gives birth to a son. She identifies the father on the birth certificate. Social services garnishes the father's wages for child support. Discuss.
2. Should the father of an unborn child have any say if the mother seeks an abortion instead of giving birth? Discuss.

Other problems in consent may arise in the case of foster children, stroke clients who cannot communicate, persons who are mentally incompetent (including those in shock and trauma), demented clients, and those temporarily or permanently under the influence of drugs or alcohol. A legal guardian who can give consent may have to be appointed by the courts. The health care staff must determine who is legally responsible in each case. When there is immediate danger to life and limb, however, the law implies consent for treatment for these individuals without consent from the responsible party.

Language can become a barrier to informed consent. An interpreter may be necessary so that information for consent can be given in a client's native tongue to ensure comprehension. If an interpreter is used, there should be a place on the consent form for the interpreter signature.

 A number of exceptions to informed consent are peculiar to each state. Examples include the following:

1. The provider may not need to disclose commonly known risks.
2. The provider may not be responsible for failing to disclose risks when the knowledge might be detrimental to the client's best interest.
3. A provider may not need to disclose risks if the client requests to remain ignorant.

A client has the right to refuse treatment. In some situations, the court appoints a guardian, who then may give consent for the client. This is especially true in the case of minors. Check your state's doctrine of informed consent for specific exceptions and information. Local medical associations also may offer information.

A unique problem surfaces for consent when the client is going to be part of any clinical trial, experimental treatment, or human research. The federal Office for Human Research Protections (OHRP), a branch of the National Institutes of Health, oversees the safety of participants in federally funded research. Each major institution that conducts research also must perform its own audit of client safety and report its results. Audits of "human subject laws," however, reveal a number of problems:

IN THE NEWS

A few states allow same sex partners to marry thereby granting the right to consent for each other. A few states are looking at legislation to allow same-sex partners many of the rights given to married couples. However, it is recommended that domestic partners who wish to consent for each other in the case of incapacity have written and notarized instructions granting the right to consent for one another.

▲ Serious adverse reactions to experimental drugs often are not recorded or reported to clients.

▲ Clients are coerced into waiving their rights to sue in case of malpractice or serious problems.

▲ Clients are placed in trials that are medically inappropriate but that needed research subjects.

▲ Informed consent is rushed due to the "desperate" nature of a participant's condition.

▲ Researchers are allowed to have financial interests in the procedures or drugs that are used, which is in direct violation of federal regulations.

▲ Not all benefits, risks, and possible alternatives are adequately explained.

OHRP records and the Food and Drug Administration (FDA) sources say the biggest problems surface at high-volume institutions where the pressure to do research is intense. Both agencies have the power to shut down clinical trials and do so; however, both agencies have limited budgets. Participation in any research places a burden on clients and their families to conduct their own investigation of the research in which they are involved.

Implementing Consent

Consent forms are prepared for the client's signature. The staff may be responsible for the preparation of specifically designed forms or the procurement of preprinted consent forms (Fig. 7–2). In either case, the form must be understandable, protect the rights of the client, and be broad enough to cover anything contemplated, but specific enough to create informed consent. A so-called "blanket consent" form, which seeks to cover all aspects of client care and is not specific, must be avoided.

Care should be given to be certain that all elements of informed consent have been understood by the client before a signature is affixed. The consent form should include an expiration date. In some states, 90 days is the maximum. Another consideration may be allowing a waiting period between consent and administration of the procedure or treatment.

The consent process ought to be concisely documented in the medical record. Some providers tape record the informed consent process and save the tapes or have a staff member present who signs the consent form also. Others have a checklist for the informed consent interview. Whatever procedures are followed, informed consent should be sought as soon as possible after the need is identified.

A health care employee may be asked to witness a signature in order to verify that the signature is indeed that of the client. The provider is responsible for the explanation of medical treatment to the client, even though the employee may provide reinforcement through clarification. If the client has any further questions about the treatment or difficulties with the consent form, let the provider know. If the client signs with an X, two witnesses are required. The younger staff members should witness consent forms; this helps ensure the longevity of the witnesses should there be any problems in later years. At least three copies of the signed consent form are necessary—one for the client, one for the medical record, and one for the hospital, if necessary.

Summary

Consent may be quite formal, requiring the signature of the client on a form that includes all the necessary components for informed consent. It may be very informal, require no formal signature, and occur in the routine activities of health care. What is most important, however, is that any consent be informed. Clients must understand and give permission for any procedures or tests to be performed. Any confusion or lack of understanding on the part of the client is an "open door" for difficulties later. Health care employees must be particularly sensitive to making certain clients comprehend what is happening.

BOTULINUM TOXIN TYPE A
(Botox Cosmetic)

Botox is made from the Botulinum Toxin Type A, a protein produced by the bacteria Clostridium botulinum. For the purpose of improving the appearance of wrinkles, small doses of the toxin are injected into the affected muscles blocking the release of a chemical that would otherwise signal the muscle to contract. The toxin thus paralyzes or weakens the injected muscle. The treatment usually begins to work within 24 to 48 hours and can last up to four months. The Food and Drug Administration (FDA) approved the cosmetic use of Botulinum Toxin Type A for the temporary relief of moderate to severe frown lines between the brow and recommends that the procedure be performed no more frequently than once every three months.

It is not known whether Botulinum Toxin Type A can cause fetal harm when administered to pregnant women or can affect reproduction capabilities. It is also not known if Botulinum Toxin Type A is excreted in human milk. For these reasons, Botulinum Toxin Type A should not be used on pregnant or lactating women for cosmetic purposes.

Patient's
Initials

_____ The details of the procedure have been explained to me in terms I understand.
_____ Alternative methods and their benefits and disadvantages have been explained to me.
_____ I understand that the FDA has only approved the cosmetic use of Botulinum Toxin Type A for frown lines between the brow. Any other cosmetic use is considered "off-label".
_____ I understand and accept the most likely risks and complications of Botulunum Toxin Type A injection(s) that include but are not limited to:

- abnormal and/or lack of facial expression
- allergic reaction/violent allergic reaction
- disorientation, double vision, and/or past pointing
- facial pain
- headache, nausea, and/or flu-like symptoms
- inability to smile when injected in the lower face
- local numbness
- paralysis of a nearby muscle, which could interfere with opening the eye(s)
- product ineffective
- temporary asymmetrical appearance
- swallowing, speech, and/or respiratory disorders
- swelling, bruising, and/or redness at injection site

_____ I understand and accept that the long-term effects of repeated use of Botox Cosmetic are as yet unknown. Possible risk and complications that have been identified include but are not limited to:

- muscle atrophy
- nerve irritability
- production of antibodies with unknown effect to general health

_____ I understand and accept that there are complications, including the remote risk of death or serious disability, that exist with this procedure.
_____ I have informed the doctor of all my known allergies.
_____ I have informed the doctor of all medications I am currently taking, including prescriptions, over-the-counter remedies, herbal therapies and supplements, aspirin, and any other recreational drug or alcohol use.
_____ I have been advised whether I should take any or all of these medications on the days surrounding the procedure.
_____ I am aware and accept that no guarantees about the results of the procedure have been made or implied.
_____ I have been informed of what to expect post treatment, including but not limited to: estimated recovery time, anticipated activity level, and the necessity of additional procedures if I wish to maintain the appearance this procedure provides me.
_____ I am not currently pregnant or nursing, and I understand that should I become pregnant while using this drug, there are potential risks, including fetal malformation.
_____ If pre- and postoperative photos and/or videos are taken of the treatment for record purposes, I understand that these photos will be the property of the attending physician.
_____ I understand that these photos may only be used for scientific or record keeping purposes.
_____ I have been advised to seek immediate medical attention if swallowing, speech, or respiratory disorders arise.
_____ The doctor has answered all of my questions regarding this procedure.

I certify that I have read and understand this treatment agreement and that all blanks were filled in prior to my signature.

I authorize and direct _____ , M.D., with associates or assistants of his or her choice, to perform the following procedure of Botulinum Toxin Type A injection(s) on _____
for the treatment of _____ .   (patient name)
                        (i.e., brow, forehead, "crow's feet," etc.)

_____   _____
Patient or Legal Representative Signature/Date   Relationship to Patient

_____   _____
Print Patient or Legal Representative Name   Witness Signature/Date

I certify that I have explained the nature, purpose, benefits, risks, complications, and alternatives to the proposed procedure to the patient. I have answered all questions fully, and I believe that the patient fully understands what I have explained.

_____
Physician Signature/ Date

_____ copy given to patient   _____ original placed in chart
 initial   initial

FIGURE 7–2 Informed consent forms: (A) for a Botulinum Toxin Type A (Botox Cosmetic) procedure (continued on page 106).

FLEXIBLE SIGMOIDOSCOPY

Flexible sigmoidoscopy involves passing a lighted flexible tube (sigmoidoscope) through the anus into the lower intestinal tract (colon). This procedure allows the practitioner to examine the inside of the lower two feet of the colon. Sometimes small tissue growths (polyps) are removed during the sigmoidoscopy (polypectomy), as polyps can grow inside the colon and become cancerous. Occasionally biopsies (sampling of small pieces of colon) are performed during the sigmoidoscopy. Bleeding sites may be treated during the sigmoidoscopy by injection of sclerosing material or use of electrocautery. On rare occasions a narrowing or obstruction may be encountered during the sigmoidoscopy. The narrowing may be stretched (dilated) at the time of sigmoidoscopy.

Patient's
Initials

____ The details of the procedure have been explained to me in terms I understand.
____ Alternative methods and their benefits and disadvantages have been explained to me.
____ I understand and accept possible risks and complications include but are not limited to:

- bleeding
- gassy discomfort/bloating
- infection
- need for surgery
- pain
- perforation

____ I have informed the doctor of all my known allergies.
____ I have informed the doctor of all medications I am currently taking, including prescriptions, over-the-counter remedies, herbal therapies and supplements, aspirin, and any other recreational drug or alcohol use.
____ I have been advised whether I should avoid taking any or all of these medications on the days surrounding the procedure.
____ I am aware and accept that no guarantees about the results of the procedure have been made.
____ I have been informed of what to expect postoperatively, including but not limited to: estimated recovery time, anticipated activity level, and the possibility of additional procedures.
____ I understand that any tissue/specimen removed during the surgery may be sent to pathology for evaluation.
____ The doctor has answered all of my questions regarding this procedure.

I certify that I have read and understand this treatment agreement and that all blanks were filled in prior to my signature.

I authorize and direct _____ , with associates or
 (practitioner's name and title, i.e., M.D., N.P., P.A.)
assistants of his or her choice, to perform a flexible sigmoidoscopy on _____.
 (patient name)

I further authorize the physician(s) and assistants to do any other procedure that in their judgment may be necessary or advisable should unforeseen circumstances arise during the procedure.

_____   _____
Patient or Legal Representative Signature/Date   Relationship to Patient

_____   _____
Print Patient or Legal Representative Name   Witness Signature/Date

I certify that I have explained the nature, purpose, benefits, risks, complications, and alternatives to the proposed procedure to the patient or the patient's legal representative. I have answered all questions fully, and I believe that the *patient/legal representative (circle one)* fully understands what I have explained.

_____
Physician Signature/ Date

____ copy given to patient   ____ original placed in chart
initial   initial

FIGURE 7–2 (continued) *(B)* For a Flexible Sigmoidoscopy surgical procedure.

Refusal to Consent to Treatment

I have been advised by Dr. _____ that the following treatment
_____ should be given to me/the below-named patient
(please type or print): _____

Dr. _____ has fully explained to me the nature and
purposes of the proposed treatment, the possible alternatives thereto and the risks
and consequences of not proceeding.

I nonetheless refuse to consent to the proposed treatment.

I have been given an opportunity to ask questions, and all my questions have
been answered to my satisfaction.

I hereby release _____ Hospital and its employees,
students and medical staff from any liability for any ill effects that I may suffer from
failure to perform the proposed treatment.

I confirm that I have read and fully understand the above and that all the
blank spaces have been completed prior to my signing.

_____   _____
Patient or Legal Guardian Signature   Date

_____   _____
Witness   Relationship

I hereby certify I have explained the nature, purpose, benefits, and alternatives
to, the proposed treatment and the risks and consequences of not proceeding,
have offered to answer any questions and have fully answered all such questions.
I believe that the patient/relative/guardian fully understands what I have explained
and answered.

_____   _____
Physician Signature   Date

Note: This document must be made part of the patient's medical records.

FIGURE 7–2 (continued) *(C)* For refusal to consent to treatment.

QUESTIONS FOR REVIEW

1. Name the difference between informed and uninformed consent.

_____

_____

2. List the four essential elements in the doctrine of informed consent.

_____

_____

3. Name two problems involved with obtaining informed consent.

_____

_____

4. The following signatures will appear on an informed consent form:

_____

_____

CLASSROOM EXERCISES

1. Jerod Hilton has just been informed that he has prostate cancer. His physician says the only course of treatment recommended is surgery. Jerod has no hesitation in his response and immediately says, "No way Doc, you aren't cutting me down there." After further discussion, Jerod's decision is unchanged. What steps, if any, does the doctor take?

2. In emergency situations, what type of consent exists? Explain and give an example.

3. The parents of a 6-year-old child consented to allow her to undergo "routine cardiac tests." One of the tests performed was a catheter arteriogram in which complications occurred. Questioning of the parents revealed that they did not fully understand the risks involved. What are the legal implications of this consent? Identify potential problems in this situation.

4. A 15-year-old enters your office requesting treatment for scalds received on his hand while emptying the dishwasher at his place of employment. Although his family receives medical treatment at your office, you are uncertain about seeing him without his parents' knowledge. Can he consent to treatment? What are the legal ramifications?

5. How specific should a consent form be? How general? Explain.

6. When you are asked to witness a signature, what does it legally mean?

7. An unmarried pregnant client requests an abortion. Assuming the abortion is legal, what rights, if any, does the father have in consent? Do you agree? Justify your reasoning.

8. After a client signed a consent form and you have witnessed it, she states, "I think this is the right decision." What would you reply? What would you do?

9. Detail what role medical assistants may assume in the consent process.

10. Refer to the vignette "When Is Enough Enough?" at the beginning of the chapter, and identify further steps that the physician might have taken to avoid the lawsuit. When *IS* enough enough?

WEB RESOURCES

▲ Physician's News Digest. "Preventing informed consent malpractice claims," by John M. Roediger, JD, April 2004. www.physiciansnews.com/law

▲ United States Department of Health and Human Services, Office for Human Research Protections (OHRP). www.hhs/gov/ohrp

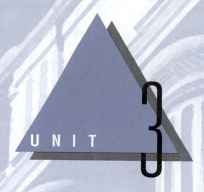

Workplace
Issues

CHAPTER 8

Medical Records

> *Do not put your faith in what statistics say until you have carefully considered what they do not say.*
>
> William W. Watt

KEY TERMS

continuous positive airway pressure (CPAP) Small electrical pump that delivers pressurized air through a nasal mask. Used to prevent airway from closing while sleeping, leading to sleep apnea.

microfiche Method of filing data on film using minute images.

problem-oriented medical record (POMR) A charting system, developed by Lawrence L. Weed, MD, that is based on client problems.

SOAP/SOAPER A charting method using subjective and objective data for client assessment and planning, education and response.

LEARNING OBJECTIVES

Upon successful completion of this chapter, you will be able to:

1. Define the key terms.
2. List six purposes of medical records in the ambulatory health care setting.
3. Name and describe two types of charting.
4. Describe *SOAP/SOAPER* and its use in medical records.

5. Demonstrate by example how and when to correct an error in medical records.
6. Discuss the impact of HIPAA on medical records.
7. Describe at least five guidelines for keeping client information private in electronic medical records and paper medical records.
8. Outline the process to follow when a subpoena or court order is received for records.
9. Explain the ownership of medical records.
10. Discuss retention and storage of medical records.

Vignette: *A day in the life of the medical record*

You are a 65-year-old female going to a large multicare health setting for an annual physical examination. When your appointment was made with the primary care physician's nurse practitioner, she noted that your physician will want fasting lab work, mammogram, and a dermatology screening. You explain that you also need a follow-up visit at the sleep clinic. All appointments are scheduled for 1 day. When you arrive, you go first to the lab for the blood draw and urinalysis. Then you have time for breakfast in the clinic's café before you see your primary care physician.

When you are in the examination room with your physician, she is able to pull the morning's lab results on her computer. She turns the computer toward you and is able to show you today's lab results on a spreadsheet with the last 2 year's results for comparison. Discussion follows. Your next stop is for a mammogram. The results of that test will be mailed to you. You hasten on to the sleep center where the physician discusses your CPAP registry that shows on his computer how many hours a night you have successfully used the breathing apparatus. He comments that your primary care physician in today's chart notes indicates that you are using a new mask and nasal pillow system that you purchased on the Internet. The final day's visit is to dermatology where you receive a full body screening for any changes in your freckles, moles, and aging spots. A suspicious mole on your lower cheek causes the dermatologist concern. She removes the mole and takes a biopsy and will notify you of the results. The dermatologist says, "I've looked at your chart; you've had a long day! Are you ready to go home now?"

The development and care of medical records require much attention from the health care staff. Both employees and physicians collect and enter data into clients' medical records. Medical records are a part of every person's life, beginning with the birth certificate and ending with the death certificate.

 The benefits of knowing your family's medical history:

▲ Better screening especially if you know someone in your family had a particular type of cancer.
▲ Better medical prevention if you are aware that someone in your family has died of a particular disease.
▲ More informed pregnancy planning that might include genetic testing and counseling if you know you have a family predisposition to some disease.
▲ Increased psychological well-being that gives you more peace of mind knowing your family history.

It is recommended that you get as much family medical information as far back as possible, at least three generations.

With increased health awareness, clients are more concerned about what goes into their medical records. Clients also care who has access to their records. Are the records legal documents? Are they confidential? What authorization is required to release clients' medical records? Who owns them? HIPAA regulations mandate that health care facilities address these questions. These are concerns health care employees face daily.

The primary goal of any medical record is the proper care and identification of the client. A client's medical record that is accurate, complete, and concise encourages better medical care than a record that is not up to date and is a folder of loose papers not necessarily related or in order.

This chapter deals with medical records in the ambulatory care setting rather than hospital medical records. Although regulations for hospital records may be mandated by state statutes and requirements for hospital licensure, regulations for medical records in the ambulatory health care setting are generally not tied to licensure; however, there are state and federal laws that pertain to ambulatory care medical records. Some facilities use the term "health" rather than "medical" records.

Purposes

The Joint Commission on Accreditation of Hospitals has established guidelines for medical records in the hospital.

 Using these as a base, the primary purposes of medical records in ambulatory health care are the following:

1. Provide a base for managing client care, which includes initiating, diagnosing, implementing, and evaluating.
2. Provide interoffice and intraoffice communication of client-related data.
3. Document total and complete health care from birth to death.
4. Allow patterns to surface that will alert physicians of clients' needs.
5. Serve as a legal basis for evidence in litigation and to protect the legal interests of clients.
6. Provide clinical data for education and research.

The medical record is an official documentation of what has happened to the client during a specific time. The type of charting and medical record used in health care settings varies. Specialists who see the client only once may have an abbreviated form of medical record. By contrast, a physician who has had the same client for 30 years may have the equivalent of three file folders with several hundred sheets of medical data on that client. Increasingly, medical charts are computerized into an electronic medical record (EMR). Whatever type is used, each client needs a medical record.

Problem-Oriented Medical Records

The **problem-oriented medical record (POMR),** or problem-oriented record (POR), was developed by Dr. Lawrence L. Weed. The POMR is based on the client's problems, and every health care employee, including the physician, adds to the chart in a particular place in the same manner. The POMR identifies the client's problems, not simply diagnoses that are based on defined data. A problem can be a condition or a behavior that results in physical or emotional distress or interferes with the client's functioning. Examples include pain in the knees and ankles, fear of falling, decreased appetite, and even an inability to pay medical bills. The problem list is usually numbered, appears on the chart face sheet, and serves as a checklist to ascertain the client's progress.

To identify clients' problems, the physician selects a database that may include a physical examination, history, laboratory tests, and subjective data from the client. Every problem has a plan, and its progress is recorded in the medical record.

Weed also developed a computerized medical record that permits the health care provider to build a computer-based POMR while accessing data pertinent to the problem from current literature.

Soap or Soaper

Many ambulatory health care settings use **SOAP/SOAPER**—subjective, objective, assessment, and plan, education, and response—as a method of charting. Once a problem is identified, it is SOAPed or SOAPERed.

▲ **Subjective** includes what the subject or client says, family comments, and hearsay; the client's exact words are recorded.

▲ **Objective** includes events that are directly observed or measurable, including laboratory tests, x-ray results, and physical examination findings.

▲ **Assessment** includes the physician's evaluation based on the subjective and objective data (S + O = A).

▲ **Plan** includes the treatment plan and the actions taken.

▲ **Education** includes any educational opportunities given.

▲ **Response** includes the client's understanding of the education and care given.

An example of the SOAP/SOAPER format is shown in Figure 8–1. SOAP/SOAPER also may be found in a source-oriented medical record, which is more likely a collection of narrative pages. Each time the client is seen by the physician, an entry is created by the physician or dictated and then transcribed by an employee. Laboratory and x-ray results are collected together; sometimes color coded, and may be shingled or layered chronologically.

Another method of narrative charting is referred to as PIE. This system of charting refers to the **p**lanning, **i**mplementation, and **e**valuation of the client's needs.

Whatever method of charting is used in medical records, it must be concise, complete, clear, and in chronological order.

CALCANEO, Henry, R. 08/18/19--

Date of Onset	Date Recorded	PROBLEMLIST	Date Resolved	INACTIVE PROBLEMS
?	10/08/2---	1. Increased appetitie, increased thirst		
			10/20/2---	
05/28/2---	06/30/2---	2. Dyspnea	07/10/2---	
05/11/2---	08/21/2---	3. Loss of job		

10/08/----

1. Increased appetite, increased thirst

S: "I eat all the time and never gain weight." "I didn't think about it, but yes, I drink water all the time, too."

O: BP 120/88. T-R-P: 98 degrees F--80--18. Color good. Skin turgor adequate. Wt. 5# less than 3 weeks ago. Urine, 4+ sugar. FBS positive.

A: Uncontrolled diabetes; in family history.

P: Dx: Lab workup for diabetes. Tx: Begin on insulin; diabetic diet.

E: Instructed to enroll, attend next diabetic class; Taught importance of diet, exercise, insulin injections. Gave our 3 clinic-prepared brochures on diabetes (intro material). Gave 24 hr phone line to call if questions.

R: Seems to understand importance of learning about diabetes, injections, diet, exercise as 2 in family have disease. Asked good questions.

07/10/----

2. Dyspnea

S: "I can't seem to get my breath. I'm weak all the time. It's worse when I lay down."

O: BP 180/98. T-R-P: 99 degrees F.--88--26. Chest x-ray negative. States he "awakens from sleep with respiratory distress." Cough; slight edema.

A: Congestive heart failure, left sided. History of hypertension and diabetes.

P: Hospitalize for cardiac workup.

E: Explain necessity of hospitalization.

R: States "I really don't want to go but if it'll help me breathe better, I'll do anything! I can't take this much more. It scares me."

07/10/----

3. Loss of Job

S: "What can I do now? I'm not trained for anything but construction, and with this heart problem and diabetes, I'll never get back my old job."

O: Heart condition improved; wt. gain 30#; brittle diabetic.

A: Is most upset that current job is not available as it's THE only job he wants. Money apparently not the issue. Off diabetic diet.

P: Return to diabetic classes w/spouse and son. Refer to Social Worker to discuss job situation.

E: Reviewed poss. complications if unsuccessful in managing his diabetes. Talked about wt gain and what it means for diabetes.

R: Good interaction w/pt; willing to attend classes w/family; concerned about complications and said he wanted to prevent any especially since one diabetic in family is nearly blind.

FIGURE 8–1 Example of a SOAP/SOAPER charting.

Legal Aspects of the Medical Record

Medical records are legal documents and as such become a vital piece of evidence in any malpractice case. Medical records that are relevant, accurate, legible, timely, informative, and complete ease the strain of any record used in litigation.

HIPAA has specific regulations about protected health information (PHI) related to electronic medical records (see Chapter 5). Under HIPAA, clients must grant written consent or permission to provide or disclose their PHI for any health care reason.

 Physicians must provide clients with a notice of their privacy practices that must include the right to:

▲ Restrict usage of PHI. This refers to the client's right to determine who has access to personal health information, how it is communicated, and what it can include.
▲ Request confidential communication. This refers to the client's right to have health information protected and kept confidential.
▲ Inspect and obtain a copy of the PHI. This refers to clients' rights to see and have a copy of their health record.
▲ Request any amendment to the PHI. This refers to clients' rights to request corrections, additions, and deletions to their health record.
▲ Receive an accounting of PHI disclosures. This refers to clients' rights to know if, when, and how their PHI and health record is disclosed.

Each state has additional and specific laws regulating the use of medical records whether or not they are electronic. For example, in Washington state, health care providers and health care facilities are required to provide a notice of information regarding the use of medical records to clients either by posting a sign or sending the notice to clients. The law further specifies what the notice must state:

> We keep a record of the health care services we provide you. You may ask us to see and copy that record. You may also ask us to correct that record. We will not disclose your record to others unless you direct us to do so or unless the law authorizes or compels us to do so. You may see your record or get more information about it at_____ . (Revised Code of Washington, a state statute, RCW 70.02.120)

Also, more states are enacting legislation regulating disclosure of information about human immunodeficiency virus (HIV) and acquired immunodeficiency syndrome (AIDS).

IN THE NEWS

HIPAA has received more than 19,000 grievances regarding alleged violations of medical privacy but Human and Health Services (HHS) has levied no civil fines and prosecuted just two criminal cases. Of the 19,420 grievances, 14,000 have either been ruled that a violation did not occur or have allowed health providers to correct violations voluntarily. At least 309 have been referred to the Department of Justice (DOJ) for possible criminal violations. The most common allegations sent to the DOJ involve improper disclosure of medical records, inadequate security for records, failure to obtain authorization to disclose records, or difficulty in patients seeking to obtain their own records.

For example, in Washington, additional consent must be obtained from the client for disclosure of HIV or AIDS information, and a court order is required to authorize disclosure of HIV information. A subpoena is not sufficient. Some states require that information related to HIV and AIDS be maintained in a special manner. Note also that a subpoena may not be sufficient to obtain other types of medical records. Substance abuse records, sexually transmitted disease records, mental health records, and sexual assault records may have explicit restrictions. Client consent or a court order may be required for such release. Health professionals should establish a protocol related to the release of medical records as well as the explicit restrictions previously mentioned.

Providers and employees should remember that the medical record might be as valuable for what it does not say as for what it does say. An act not recorded is generally considered an act not performed by most courts of law. The necessity of using a medical record in a court emphasizes the importance of accurate records that honestly reflect the client's course of treatment. Also, some clinics do periodic audits of their charts to ensure good charting practices.

If an error is made on a medical record, it must be properly corrected. Handwritten errors discovered later should be corrected by the following method: draw a line through the error using a red pen, write "correction" or "corr.," sign your initials, indicate the date, and write in the correction. An electronic error is made much the same way. Using the tracking device in the word processing software, a line is drawn through the error. The correction is then placed right after the information lined out and the words "correction" or "corr" are indicated as well as your initials and the date the correction is made. When erasures or obliterations occur, confusion and suspicion may result. Poor or altered records can be detrimental to the physician's defense in court.

The medical record often becomes the center of a malpractice action wherein both attorneys involved will bring in forensic document examiners to investigate the reliability of the record. Such experts will use specialized equipment that can detect different inks in the same entry, a fact that a jury could easily interpret to be an indication of the record having been tampered with. Scientific equipment also can detect when pages have been added after the fact. Health professionals should never change a medical record unless correcting it properly. Never "leave room" for someone else to chart later. Such a space may cause suspicion. Finally, never remove a report or note from a medical record because it, too, may indicate that a record has undergone tampering.

The medical record is confidential. HIPAA as well as state regulations require employees handling records to protect the privacy of clients unless otherwise mandated by law. Some states consider communication between client and physician to be privileged. The privilege belongs to clients and is important because physicians need to know highly personal and private information about clients during the course of treatment.

No information is released from the medical record without the physician's approval and the written permission of the client, and then only the specific information authorized is released (Fig. 8-2). Creating a form that may be signed by clients for the release of any med-

---

IN THE NEWS

According to a Cincinnati Children's Hospital Medical Center study, verbal medical orders have been reduced from a 9.1 percent error rate to zero simply by having residents read back the order for the attending physician's verification, before entering it into the computer. Although the sample was small (75 orders), it has implications for other health care settings besides the hospital.

ical records may be helpful. The simplest release is seen on many insurance claim forms, which require the client's signature before certain data are released to the insurance carrier.

If the client is a minor, the parent or legal guardian may sign. If the parents are legally separated or divorced, the parent who has legal custody of the minor must sign all release forms. If the client is incompetent, the court-appointed guardian signs the release of information. If the client is deceased, the legal representative of the estate signs the release form. Recent laws have allowed some government and state agencies, such as those that administer the Medicare and Medicaid program, access to medical records without clients' consent. A standard procedure is essential for maintaining confidentiality and good client relations.

At times during the course of medical practice a court order or a subpoena may be received requesting a client's medical chart and/or specific information from the chart. Notify the client prior to releasing the record in accordance with the subpoena. In some states, the attorney who subpoenas the medical record must notify in writing both the provider and the

AUTHORIZATION TO RELEASE INFORMATION

Please Print Clearly

Name _____
              (Last)   (First)   (M.I.)

Address _____
              (Street)   (City)   (State)

Phone (_____)_____ Date of Birth_____ Medical Record #_____
I authorize_____ to release medical information from my medical record to
Name of Doctor, Hospital, etc. _____
Address _____
City/State/Zip Code_____

for the purpose of review/examination. I further authorize you to provide such copies thereof as may be requested.
The foregoing is subject to such limitation as indicated below:
☐ Entire record
☐ Specific information:_____
☐ Old records from previous physicians:_____

I give special permission to release any information regarding: (initial on applicable line(s) below)

_____ Substance Abuse _____ Psychiatric/Mental Health Information _____ HIV Information

Reason for request_____
This authorization will automatically expire 90 days from the date signed. I understand that I may revoke this
content at any time except to the extent that action has been taken in reliance thereon.

Signed _____ Date _____

Witness _____ Date _____

FOR OFFICE USE ONLY

Received_____ Completed By_____
Completed _____ Fee Paid_____
Amount Billed $_____ Amount Due _____

Disclosure Consisted Of _____
_____
_____
_____
_____

Name

FIGURE 8–2 Sample of a form authorizing the release of information.

Date: _____
RE: _____
History #/Date of Birth _____

This is a multiple action form letter with only those items indicated by an "X" being applicable.

IN ANSWER TO YOUR REQUEST FOR MEDICAL INFORMATION

Please see attached medical record copies. NOTE: Request for copies of the entire record will include only the last 2 years of lab work. The attached medical information is CONFIDENTIAL. Subsequent disclosure is not authorized without the specific consent of the patient.

REQUEST FOR ADDITIONAL INFORMATION

☐ Your request is being returned for the following reason(s):

    ☐ We are unable to locate a record of treatment for this individual. Please provide additional information, such as full name of patient at time of treatment, date of birth, history #, or verification of spelling of name. RETURN YOUR REQUEST WITH THE INFORMATION.

    ☐ No record on file for specified dates.

    ☐ Medical information is confidential and can be released only on written consent of patient /patient's legally authorized representative. HAVE THE PATIENT COMPLETE THE ENCLOSED CONSENT AND RETURN YOUR REQUEST WITH THE CONSENT.

    ☐ Authorization date is over 6 months. RETURN YOUR REQUEST WITH A MORE RECENTLY DATED AUTHORIZATION SIGNED BY THE PATIENT/PATIENT'S LEGALLY AUTHORIZED REPRESENTATIVE.

    ☐ The authorization received contained insufficient information for release of the information requested.

☐ Our charge for releasing records directly to the patient/patient's representative is $_____ . If you provide us with the name and address of your new physician, we will send the copies there instead, thereby eliminating the charge. Otherwise, make check payable to_____put patient's name on the check, and return a copy of this letter with check.

☐ Please remit _____, which is our fee for processing your request and photocopying the requested record. Make check payable to_____, reference the patient's name on the check, and return a copy of this letter with check.

☐ Other: _____
_____
_____
_____
_____
_____

FIGURE 8–2 (continued)

client and allow 14 days for a response. Unless the original is subpoenaed, a certified photocopy should be made for the courts. If the original is subpoenaed, a copy should be made to remain in the office. An original medical record should be hand delivered to the court clerk and a receipt obtained. The person or agency issuing the subpoena usually pays the cost of making copies.

▲ CRITICAL THINKING EXERCISE

1. The medical assistant is catching up on the completeness of the practice's medical records. She notices that the physician wants a transcript of two telephone calls that had not been previously recorded. She now records them, post dates when the calls were made, and signs the entry. Discuss.
2. A well-informed client discusses her marital problems with the physician, and says, "Please do not put this in my record." Discuss.

Electronic Medical Records

HIPAA requires standardization of electronic patient health data and security standards to protect the confidentiality and integrity of the individually identifiable health information past, present, or future. Facilities must make certain their computers containing confidential information about clients are protected.

The following guidelines are important.

▲ Computer hardware, servers, and network hubs are to be kept secure from intrusion.
▲ A list of users approved to access medical information must be identified and regularly updated.
▲ Robust firewalls and anti-virus measures must be in place. Blocking of unauthorized intrusion must be in place.
▲ Passwords are to be changed at least every 90 days, and created so they are not easily guessed.
▲ Passwords are hidden when entered and are securely stored. They are not to be shared with anyone.
▲ The computer station should limit the number of invalid attempts to access information.
▲ Computer screens are to be out of view of the public and unauthorized staff.
▲ Screensavers should be used to prevent unwanted viewers' access.

Ideally, any time a computer workstation is vacated, even for a short period, the user should close out of the document, allowing the screen saver to activate. Upon returning, the user would again need to enter the protected password for access to the medical information.

When a paper medical record is used, the same careful attention needs to be paid to keeping clients' health care information private. If not in a private area, turn over any pieces of paper that might be viewed by another individual. Never leave a medical record unattended or open in any workspace. Make certain that a client's name cannot be read by outsiders on the chart face or index tab. Keep in mind that this kind of information is protected from unauthorized access. This may require the storage of all medical charts in an enclosed and locked cabinet so that even housekeepers are not able to see any personal data regarding clients.

If the health facility also contracts with other business associates, they, too, must comply and ensure their compliance to HIPAA. For example, each entity needs to use safeguards to prevent disclosure of PHI, to provide an accounting of any disclosures, and to return or destroy the PHI at termination of their services or contract. It is the hiring health facility that needs to ensure that its contracted businesses follow HIPAA guidelines.

Not all health care clinics are computerized; however, computerized records allow health care professionals to remind clients of appointments and, in many cases, to track client progress faster and more easily. Less storage space is necessary for computerized files, and files can be more easily retrieved. In some cases, the computerized charts are less likely to be misplaced. Of course, files can be easily deleted from the computer. Therefore, written procedures are to be established for adding to or changing data on the computer, including who is authorized to make changes, the time in which changes can take place, and who will be informed of those changes. Procedures need to be developed for purging aged data.

E-Mail

E-mail is a useful tool for the health care setting. It provides communication among providers and their employees, and between provider and client. It creates a written record that information was shared, allows embedding of educational links, and can be used in malpractice suits to exhibit communication. However, e-mail has its disadvantages. Namely, e-mail is not a private or confidential means of communication; it is discoverable even after deleting; it may be necessary to obtain consent before sending; e-mail may be misread and misunderstood; e-mail can be monitored, accessed, and read by supervisors without liability for privacy invasion; and e-mail is the property of the agency/facility. See Figure 8–3 for sample email and fax confidentiality statements.

HIPAA requires specific consent for any electronic mail transmission of PHI.

If e-mail is used in your practice, the following guidelines should be followed:

1. Establish time lines for reading and responding to e-mail.
2. Generate automated replies to acknowledge you have received e-mail.
3. Inform clients of the privacy risks of using e-mail.
4. Do not use e-mail without informed consent.
5. Avoid using e-mail that requires an urgent reply.
6. Place e-mail correspondence in client records and ensure the e-mails are properly identified.
7. Do not forward e-mail without permission.
8. Ensure that no one else has access to your e-mail account and do not leave your monitor unattended while signed onto your e-mail account.
9. Establish specific procedures for personal digital assistant (PDA) devices if they carry e-mail and client information.
10. Frequently change passwords.
11. Have staff sign confidentiality contracts.

▲ CRITICAL THINKING EXERCISE

A client e-mails her internist requesting permission to begin a water therapy class at the local YMCA that requires a physician's release. The internist responds to the e-mail within 24 hours and says, "Sounds like a good plan. Fax me the release form." The client faxes the release form to the physician's clinic. He completes it and faxes it directly to the therapist at the YMCA. Discuss the advantages of this activity to the client and to the internist. Does it raise any problems?

Fax Machines

The facsimile (fax) machine can be especially useful if health care information is needed more quickly than can be accomplished by mail, phone, or computer. Also, more detail can be given by fax than by phone. There are problems, however. The fax may inadvertently be sent to the wrong destination or retrieved by an unauthorized recipient. Therefore, careful attention to confidentiality must be considered when using a fax transmission for client medical records. (See Figure 8–3.) Office policies should be initiated detailing proper procedures.

Use the following fax guidelines:

1. Use the fax machine only when there is not enough time for more secured measures such as mailing.
2. Use the fax machine only when machines are located in restricted–access, secure areas.
3. Obtain appropriate client authorization where required before the release of information.
4. Verify the recipient of the fax, the fax number, and the location of the fax machine. Include a statement to those who might receive the fax in error. Call to see if the fax was received.
5. Document the reason for any fax transmission and any misdirected fax.

Figure 8–3 illustrates a sample confidentiality notice to accompany any e-mail or fax.

> **Confidentiality Notice**: This message and any attachments may contain confidential and privileged communications or information. The information contained in this e-mail/fax is transmitted for the sole use of the intended recipient(s). The authorized recipient of this e-mail/fax is prohibited from disclosing this information to any other party. If you are not the intended recipient or designated agent of the recipient of such information, you are hereby notified that any use, dissemination, copying or retention of this e-mail/fax or the information contained herein is strictly prohibited. If you received this e-mail/fax in error, please notify the sender immediately and permanently delete this e-mail/fax.

FIGURE 8–3 Confidentiality notice.

Ownership of Medical Records

The accepted rule is that medical records are the property of the person or persons entering the data in them. Physicians are considered the owners of the medical records they have written. However, clients have access to the information in their medical records. Clients may be expected to make an appointment to obtain that copy and pay reproduction fees. Access should be withheld only when the law prohibits such access, or when, in the physician's opinion, great harm would be done to the client.

Clients who request that their medical records be transferred to another physician must do so in writing. The original record may be retained in the office and the request honored with a photocopy of the complete record or the physician's summary. The continuance of medical records is important in a society that is so mobile. This continuity can be accomplished only with cooperation from physicians. The important factor is to release the record promptly so that the client can receive proper care from the new physician.

▲ CRITICAL THINKING EXERCISE

1. The use of "smart cards" has been suggested as a remedy for protecting clients' medical information. The encoded smart card contains a person's medical record and only that person releases the information contained therein by sharing a personally chosen password. Discuss the advantages/disadvantages of such a system.
2. Would you prefer regular e-mail access or telephone access for your primary care provider? Explain your answer.

Retention of Medical Records

The question of how long to retain medical records is not easily answered. One guideline indicates that records should be retained until the statute of limitations for acts of medical malpractice has expired so that records are available for any possible litigation. This guideline may require a pediatrician to keep the record for as long as 7 to 10 years beyond the age of maturity.

REMEMBER... Physicians probably should keep clients' medical records permanently. However, keeping medical records for 7 to 15 years after clients are no longer seeing the physician or 5 years after the date of last service for deceased clients is probably sufficient.

Storage of Medical Records

Not all paper medical records need to be kept in the same location. Active records should be in readiness for physicians. Closed or inactive files usually include records of clients who are no longer being seen by the physician, who may have moved away, or who have died. These files may be kept in a storage area separate from the current and active files. The office may have storage space or may rent storage space in another location. Files may be stored on **microfiche** and, if so, will require a reader in order to access the information. In today's computerized society, medical records are most likely stored electronically and will not pose such a serious storage problem. These stored records need to be protected as carefully as active files.

Summary

Medical records carry pertinent client information and data that, in part, determine the care given. Medical records have very sensitive information, must be kept private and confidential, and any information released must be done so only with the consent of the client and/or a "medical need to know" basis. Health care professionals must always remember that medical records may become a critical document in litigation of what was or was not performed. Well thought out documentation in medical records that is complete, organized, sequential, and kept confidential and private tell a story of meticulous client care.

QUESTIONS FOR REVIEW

1. Name four purposes of the medical record.

_____

_____

2. Explain how POMR is used.

_____

_____

3. SOAP/SOAPER means

_____

_____

4. The health care employee needs to remember the following to prepare a medical record that will be a good defense in a lawsuit:

_____

_____

5. Telecommunication by computer, e-mail, and fax should be used in the following manner:

_____

_____

6. The following person(s) own(s) the medical record:

_____

_____

7. A medical record should be retained for the following length of time:

_____

_____

CLASSROOM EXERCISES

1. A fax was received in a private home. The resident was not expecting a fax. When she picks it up, she sees it comes from a nearby long-term-care facility, is addressed to a physician, has personal information about a resident of the facility, and requests a medication change. What should the owner do? What responsibility and action does the long-term facility take?

2. While you are preparing the client for the physician, the client picks up the medical record and begins to read it. What do you do?

3. The following report was phoned in and charted: "Urinalysis 09/16/0– reveals RBC too numerous to count." When the written report is received, you note it as WBC, not RBC. Properly correct.

4. You are preparing a medical record after it has been subpoenaed. Describe the procedures you would follow. What do you do with medical information from a referring physician?

5. A client becomes angry when refused permission to hand carry medical records when moving out of state. What alternatives can an employee suggest?

6. Describe what might be done when there is simply no room for any more medical records in the office.

7. Refer to the vignette "A Day in the Life of the Medical Record." As a client, how did the availability of the medical record facilitate the care received? As a health care provider, what are the advantages of having up-to-the-minute information on the client? Discuss the legal implications of a medical record used in this manner.

WEB RESOURCES

▲ HIPAA Advisory. www.hipaadvisory.com

▲ Journal of Medical Internet Research. "Doctors Who Are Using E-mail With Their Patients: a Qualitative Exploration," by Madhavi R. Patt, Thomas K. Houston, Mollie W. Jenckes, Daniela Z Sands, and Daniel E. Ford. www.jmir.org

▲ Journal of Medical Internet Research. "Providing a Web-based Online Medical Record with Electronic Communication Capabilities to Patients With Congestive Health Failure: Randomized Trial," by Stephan E. Ross, Laurie A. Moore, Mark A. Earnest, Loretta Wittevrongel. www.jmir.org

▲ Med League Support Services, Inc. "Medical Errors and Litigation: Investigation and Case Preparation," edited by Jon R. Abele, Esq. www.medleague.com

CHAPTER 9

Reimbursement and Collection Practices

> *Even if you're on the right track, you'll get run over if you just sit there.*
>
> *Will Rogers*

KEY TERMS

capitation Physicians are paid a fixed monthly fee for a range of services for each HMO member in their care.

co-payment A medical expense that is a member's responsibility; usually a fixed amount of $5 to $20.

COBRA Consolidated Omnibus Budget Reconciliation Act of 1985 mandates that continuation of group insurance coverage be offered to covered persons who lose health or dental coverage due to a qualifying event.

deductible A cost-sharing arrangement in which the member pays a set amount toward covered services before the insurer begins to make any payments. Typically, HMO members do not pay deductibles.

diagnostic related group (DRG) A classification system that groups together patients who are similar in their diagnosis and treatment, and in their consumption of hospital resources, thus allowing comparisons of resource use across hospitals with varying mixes of patients. Used primarily in the United States as a method of funding hospitals.

health maintenance organization (HMO) Prepaid health care services rendered by participating physicians and providers to an enrolled group of persons.

independent practice association (IPA) Is an entity that offers a number of reimbursement plans and contracts with providers who practice independently in their own clinics.

International Classification of Diseases, 10th revision, Clinical Modifications (ICD-10-CM) Listing that identifies the diagnostic categories, specific DRG numbers, and monetary values. That monetary value is how United States hospitals and providers are reimbursed unless there are extenuating circumstances.

managed care A type of health care plan; generally one of two types, namely HMO or preferred provider organization (PPO).

medical savings accounts (MSA) A method for companies with 50 or fewer employees, self-employed persons, and the uninsured to purchase medical insurance by making tax-free deposits to an MSA.

pay for performance (P4P) A type of managed care that encourages physicians to improve the quality of their clients' care, and reimburses them for their progress toward a fixed goal.

preferred provider organization (PPO) A type of business agreement between a medical service provider and an insurer organization in which the fees for specific services are predetermined for an already established group of clients assigned to or selected by the provider.

primary care physician (PCP) A physician in an HMO who authorizes medical care to clients.

usual, customary, and reasonable fee (UCR) Describes how providers are reimbursed for their services and is widely accepted by insurance carriers. The usual fee is a provider's average fee for a service or what is usually charged for a procedure. The customary fee is the average of fees within a particular geographical area for a described service or procedure and performed by the same kind of provider. The reasonable fee is what is normally acceptable for services that are unusually difficult or complicated.

LEARNING OBJECTIVES

Upon successful completion of this chapter, you will be able to:

1. Define key terms.
2. Explain, in a short paragraph, the importance of appropriate reimbursement and collections.
3. List at least five guidelines related to reimbursement.
4. Recall the laws that have an impact on reimbursement.
5. Describe five government insurance programs.
6. Discuss the suggestions that help clients be financially responsible for their health care.
7. List at least five items to be covered in a collection policy.
8. Identify the appropriate procedures to follow when collecting a bill by telephone or by mail.
9. Identify the seven "collection don'ts" established by the Federal Trade Commission.
10. Address solutions to collections problems.
11. Explain the one important procedure to follow if a client is denied credit because of a poor credit rating.
12. List steps to follow in selecting a collection agency.
13. Discuss ethical implications regarding reimbursement and collections.

Vignette: Can you afford this?

A general surgeon practicing in a metropolitan area loves his work. He spends only 1 day of the week in the clinic and performs about six operations a week. He no longer covers night emergencies. Early in his practice, he determined that insurance companies were totally dictating his compensation so he quit accepting any insurance. To see this general surgeon, clients must pay cash. If clients want to file for reimbursement from their insurer, it is up to them. His fees are based on what the market will bear. His net income for at least a decade has been nearly 1.2 million dollars per year.

Physicians and health care providers will receive reimbursement for their services from many different sources. Successful practice management, billing, and collections require knowledgeable personnel who understand the complex characteristics of how reimbursement is made. Clients receiving care have many options for making payments. Sixty years ago, clients expected to pay physicians the full fee for services at the time they were rendered. Out of courtesy, some physicians would send a statement at the end of the month. Insurance of any kind was rare.

Today, physicians may be paid any of the following ways: (1) Payment received through a client's insurance plan, probably receiving only a percentage of allowable charges; (2) Is likely paid according to a rate established by a predetermined **diagnostic related group** (DRG); (3) May receive only a set fee for a client in a **capitation** arrangement no matter what the costs were; (4) May receive payment from credit and debit cards; (5) May be paid a bonus if they perform well in giving service across a spectrum of quality measures (**Pay for Performance or P4P**; see Chapter 2); (6) May receive payment through an automatic-payment program where an insurance carrier has permission to make payroll deductions from served clients; (7) Cash received for full or partial payment. The complexity of medical reimbursement has created a bookkeeping/accounting nightmare for health care providers. The most successful facilities in the arena of reimbursement likely have at least one individual, many times several, whose sole responsibility is payment and collections. They have computerized their billing, and spend at least a couple of hours weekly in appealing denied insurance claims.

 There are a number of guidelines to keep in mind related to client reimbursement. They include, but are not limited to, the following:

▲ Help clients understand their medical services and how much they cost.
▲ Provide cost estimates as often as possible so clients know what to expect.
▲ Expect to explain to clients at least the basic principles of insurance reimbursement according to their individual plan.
▲ Clearly identify what clients are expected to pay and when.
▲ Never bill for a service that is not clearly identified and appropriately charted.
▲ Carefully adhere to all laws pertaining to reimbursement and collections.
▲ Establish a reimbursement and collections policy.
▲ Treat all clients equitably and fairly and without regard for their financial status.

However billing and collections is accomplished, there are numerous legal aspects to consider. A brief presentation of applicable laws for reimbursement and collections is given. Ethical concerns are addressed later in this chapter.

Laws for Reimbursement and Collections

Truth in Lending Act

Regulation Z of the Consumer Protection Act of 1968 is also known as the Truth in Lending Act. This act is enforced by the Federal Trade Commission, and when applied to the health care setting deals with collection of clients' payments.

Briefly, the regulation requires that an agreement by providers and their clients for payment of medical bills in more than four installments must be in writing and must provide information regarding finance charges. Even if no finance charge is involved, the agreement must be in writing and stipulate no finance charge.

If consumers decide to pay their bills by installments unilaterally with no established agreement with providers, Regulation Z is not applicable as long as the provider continues to bill for the full amount.

Situations in which the Truth in Lending Act is often used include arrangements for surgery, prenatal or delivery care for fee-for-service plans or other medical services not covered by insurance. The amount owed by the client is often more than a client can pay in one installment or is more than is covered by medical insurance. Health care employees then can discuss with the client appropriate installment payments, put the agreement in writing, and provide a copy for the client. Few providers will charge a finance fee in this situation, although to do so is both legal and ethical. If bilateral installment agreements are common or if computer billing automatically includes a finance charge after a certain period, have the wording approved by a legal representative.

Truth in Lending Consumer Credit Loss Disclosure is similar to the Truth in Lending Act but goes a step further. It requires providers to disclose all additional costs such as interest and late charges and to include them on the billing statement.

The Equal Credit Opportunity Act

The Equal Credit Opportunity Act ensures that all consumers are given an equal chance to obtain credit so when providers extend credit for one client, all clients must be offered the same opportunity. Providers may deny credit to clients based on their inability to pay and inform their clients that credit has been denied. Clients then have 60 days to request the rationale for the denial in writing.

Fair Credit Billing Act

The Fair Credit Billing Act states that clients have 60 days to complain about any error in their billing. The health care employee must document, acknowledge the complaint, and respond within 90 days to the complaint. The response may be to correct any error or to explain to the client why the bill was accurate.

Fair Debt Collections Practices Act

The Fair Debt Collections Practices Act, a federal law governed by the Federal Trade Commission, addresses the communication that occurs when collecting debts in the manner a collections agency might. According to the law, its purpose is to eliminate abusive debt collection practices by debt collectors, to ensure that those debt collectors who refrain from using abusive debt collection practices are not competitively disadvantaged, and to promote consistent state action to protect consumers against debt collection abuses.

Federal Wage Garnishing Law

The Federal Wage Garnishing Law addresses payment of debts utilizing employee salaries. Garnishment means to attach a person's property or wages by court order to pay debts. The law limits the amount of money that can be garnished and protects an employee from being dismissed because of garnishment. Federal employees, however, are exempt from this law. Some state laws may differ from the federal law so it is best for the health care professional to contact either the Department of Labor or legal counsel for clarification. Garnishment of salary is one method that can be used to collect a fairly large delinquent account.

Tax Equity Fiscal Responsibility Act

The Tax Equity Fiscal Responsibility Act is a federal law that addresses hospitalization payments for Medicare. It specifies provisions relating to savings in health and income security programs. This includes changes in payment for services, benefits, and premiums of Medicare as well as changes in provisions under Medicaid and other specific programs covered by Social Security.

The prospective payment system using Diagnosis Related Groups (DRG) reimburses hospitals on a lump sum rather than a fee-for-service basis. DRGs classify clients who are medically related according to diagnosis, treatment, and length of hospital stay. **The International Classification of Diseases, 10th revision, Clinical Modifications** (ICD-10-CM) identifies the diagnostic categories, specific DRG numbers, and monetary values. That monetary value is how United States hospitals and providers are reimbursed unless there are extenuating circumstances. The role of the health professional is important in this type of reimbursement because the initial hospitalization diagnosis generally comes from the admitting physician who is in ambulatory care.

Stark I and II Regulations

Stark I and II Regulations prohibit a physician or provider from referring a Medicare client for services to an entity with which the physician or immediate family member has a financial relationship through ownership or compensation, unless the referral is protected by one or more exceptions provided in the law. For details of the Stark I and II Regulations, it is imperative that health professionals review information found in the Federal Registry.

Civil Monetary Penalties Act

The Civil Monetary Penalties Act addresses Medicare and Medicaid fraud and provides for prosecution in such cases. Physicians or providers who falsely bill clients' services or incorrectly code services can be liable for their acts under this regulation. Hence, health care employees must be current in Medicare and Medicaid policies and be honest in their coding and billing procedures.

Deficit Reduction Act

The Deficit Reduction Act was enacted in 1984 and revised in 2005. It addresses Medicare reimbursement by increasing physician and provider service payment rates to the 2005 level. In ensuing years, the health professional will see continuing adjustments in Medicare rates. Overall, the 2005 Act was enacted to address the Medicare program and provider reimbursement without cutting services to clients.

How Physicians Are Paid

Usual, customary, and reasonable fee (UCR) describes how providers are reimbursed for their services. The usual fee is a provider's average fee for a service or what is usually charged for a procedure. The customary fee is the average of fees within a particular geographical area for a described service or procedure and performed by the same kind of provider. The reasonable fee is what is normally acceptable for services that are unusually difficult or complicated. The UCR is widely accepted across the country by insurance carriers, and provides a basis for reimbursement to providers.

IN THE NEWS

Ho Ling Lai of Framingham, Massachusetts, pleaded guilty July 18, 2006 before U.S. District Judge Reginald C. Lindsay to knowingly and willfully committing health care fraud. Lai, a physical therapist working for three different nurse associations, billed Medicare for physical therapy services to a patient of each of the nurse associations at the same time, on the same day, but in different towns. Medicare was falsely billed for $55,000. Lai faced a maximum sentence of 10 years in prison and a $250,000 fine.

Private pay may come from clients who have no work-related medical insurance, insufficient medical insurance, and/or do not qualify for any government health care coverage. These clients may be working only part-time, never having enough hours to qualify for insurance benefits, or they may choose a medical service that is not covered by insurance. Payment is usually made at the time of service unless other arrangements are made.

Individual policies are a kind of personal insurance. Clients may have to submit to a physical examination and give a detailed medical history to qualify. Premiums are generally expensive and benefits may be less than other plans.

Group policies are designed for a group of individuals covered under a master contract issued to their employer. Both employers and employees pay a percentage of the premiums. Deductions may be made from salaries to help pay the costs of group plans. Premiums are less costly than individual policies, and benefits are greater. A physical examination is not normally required.

Government plans include the following:

▲ Civilian Health and Medical Program of the Uniformed Services (CHAMPUS) was formed in 1956 to provide medical treatment to authorized dependents of military personnel. Since 1994, CHAMPUS is known as TRICARE. TRICARE covers family members of active duty personnel; military retirees and their eligible members under the age of 65, and spouses, if unmarried; and children, if unmarried survivors of all uniformed services. The program is managed by the military in concert with civilian hospitals and clinics. CHAMPVA was formed in 1973 to provide benefits to dependents of veterans. In some instances, if the client has other insurance coverage, health care professionals will bill that insurance as well.

▲ Medicaid, in 1965, made agreements with states to provide health care to the medically indigent. The federal government provides funds to the states that, in turn, decide how to use those funds in providing medical care. Medicaid also covers certain individuals receiving federal and state aid, persons who receive supplemental Social Security payments, recipients of Aid to Families with Dependent Children, pays Medicare premiums for some low-income elderly, and provides **COBRA** coverage for low-income persons who lose employer health insurance benefits.

▲ Medicare is a federal insurance program established in 1966 for people 65 years of age or older, for individuals who are blind or disabled, and for people on kidney dialysis or who have had a kidney transplant. There are two parts to this plan: Part A is hospital insurance and requires no premiums from clients; Part B is medical insurance and requires a monthly premium. As of January, 2006, Medicare D provided everyone with Medicare access to prescription drug coverage. There is a range of plans available for Part D, all requiring a premium to be paid by recipients.

▲ Workers' Compensation programs were established in all states to cover the cost of medical care resulting from accident or illness related to a person's employment. Loss of income benefits are also included. The provider of services must accept the workers' compensation as payment in full and cannot bill the client.

Managed Care Plans provide health care within a network of providers for a predetermined and set fee. The Health Maintenance Organization Act of 1973 defined the characteristics of managed care. Managed care insurance plans attempt to reduce costs by limiting where and from whom clients can receive medical services. Some plans limit any type of specialty care. Managed care is given via numerous models:

▲ *Health Maintenance Organizations* **(HMO)** are prepaid health care services rendered by participating physicians or providers to an enrolled group of persons. An HMO comes in a number of differing forms. The *prepaid group practice* occurs when providers form their own group and contract with an HMO to provide medical services to enrolled members. A *staff* HMO is owned by the HMO and pays providers a salary. A **Primary Care Provider (PCP)** authorizes medical care. An *independent practice association (IPA)* does not maintain its own staff and buildings. It contracts with providers practicing independently in their own offices and clinics, and offers a number of reimbursement plans. HMO payment plans may include some form of capitation, P4P, or bonus for successful providers.

▲ **Preferred Provider Organization (PPO)** is a form of managed care where providers agree upon a predetermined set of charges for all services provided. Clients will have **deductibles** and coinsurance responsibilities; the PPO pays for the remaining balance.

There are other methods in which providers may receive reimbursement. Clients who have long-term-care insurance may be able to use a portion of those benefits to pay medical bills, especially if they have a life-threatening illness. Some life insurance policies allow clients to draw from the policy benefit to pay medical indebtedness. Disability insurance, whether or not work-related, can be used to pay for related medical expenses. **Medical savings accounts (MSA)** provide a method for companies with 50 or fewer employees, self-employed persons, and the uninsured to purchase medical insurance by making tax-free deposits to an MSA. Clients can use the funds in their MSA to pay for routine medical expenses. Any money in the account at the end of the year earns tax-free interest.

Clients' Responsibility for Reimbursement

With or without the involvement of an insurance plan for health care costs, clients are still responsible for the payment of their medical bills. There are a number of suggestions to help clients be responsible and to make billing and collections less complex for ambulatory health care employees.

REMEMBER...

▲ Request payment for any coinsurance, deductibles, or exclusions at the time of service.
▲ If there is no insurance, expect payment at the time of service, and offer installment payments if necessary.
▲ Provide clients a detailed analysis of the services provided and the charges. You cannot expect payment up front if clients have not been provided this information.
▲ Offer debit/credit card payment for services provided. Remember that you cannot charge clients the fees the facility pays for the use of debit/credit cards.
▲ If clients are to be denied services because of inability to pay, offer and discuss alternatives.

Collection Guidelines

Collection procedures may be necessary to obtain full payment of services provided to clients. Collection procedures must be firm but temperate enough not to irritate otherwise satisfied consumers who intend to pay. If they feel comfortable doing so, providers should not hesitate to discuss directly with consumers the fees for their services. Many times, a client more readily accepts a statement of fees from a doctor than from an employee.

Medical managers must establish an appropriate collection policy for employees to follow (Box 9–1). Clients need to be informed in writing of the policy. That policy should state how insurance claims are handled. Will the office file claims for all insurance carriers, or only a certain few? Does the client in a managed care plan ever receive a bill; if so, under what circumstances? The policy should state how and when **co-payments** and deductibles are collected. The policy should determine whether and at what point collection letters will be sent. Will there be a minimum payment schedule? Will the collection letter be different for every account? Are collection telephone calls to be made; if so, by whom? How many?

B O X   9.1   **Collecting Fees**

Establishing a good procedure for collecting fees can eliminate headaches later.

▲ Establish fees
▲ Discuss fees
▲ Have a written fee policy
▲ Expect payment at time of service
▲ Provide a policy brochure
▲ Ask for payment before client leaves the office
▲ Provide a stamped, addressed envelope for payment
▲ Send accurate, itemized statements
▲ Have a follow-up policy
▲ Have a collection agency policy

When? What procedures will be followed? Will delinquent accounts ever be turned over to a collection agency or pursued through the local courts? A clearly defined or stated policy gives employees the support necessary for successful collections.

It is important to build a professional and cooperative relationship with insurers to prevent billing problems and delayed or inaccurate reimbursements. Medical personnel should meet periodically with insurance representatives to learn their rules and billing processes. When specific problems arise, discuss with representatives and pose possible solutions. Ask for definite solutions to be put in writing. Gather and analyze your computerized payment records and identify those insurers who are chronically late with payments. Then use this with the insurer to negotiate a better reimbursement time line. Clinics have a right to reimbursement within 90 days on accurately submitted bills.

Collection Do's

The following guidelines are provided to suggest possible procedures for collections in the health care setting:

1. Establish appropriate fees for the services.
2. Discuss fees with consumers the first time they present themselves or call for treatment. A written payment policy is essential. Explain to consumers their responsibilities in a managed care plan.
3. Expect clients to pay any co-payments, deductibles, or exclusions at the time of service.
4. Provide clients with an office brochure that gives them information about hours, emergency contacts, physicians' or providers' services, how billing is handled, and whom to call if there is a question about a bill. Identify the insurances accepted by the providers.
5. Provide an opportunity for the client to pay their responsibility before leaving the office. The charge slip or encounter form is an ideal way for the provider to indicate charges and services, as well as the diagnoses. The bill is then presented to clients, who are asked to stop at the receptionist's desk on their way out. The receptionist can say, "Mrs. Lotta M. Bucks, your charge today is $165. Would you like to pay by cash, check, debit or credit card?" Some clinics have been successful in providing clients with a stamped, addressed envelope in which to mail the fee when they return home or are billed at the end of the month.
6. Have an established practice for mailing statements, and follow that practice. Statements should be itemized, accurate, and easy to understand. Make sure all credits have been

posted up to the closing date. They should be mailed to arrive the first of the month. Statements that include envelopes, especially colored ones, are paid faster.

7. When your collection policy dictates that a bill should be followed with a letter or a telephone call, do it. Be consistent, pleasant, and firm. The sooner you follow through on a delinquent account, the more likely it will be collected.

8. Employees responsible for collections should have certain phrases and the wording of possible letters at their fingertips for quick and easy referral. They also need the authority to carry the collection process to its completion.

9. Suggested procedures for mail or telephone collections include the following: (a) Introduce yourself. (b) Establish that you are speaking to the proper person, if it is a telephone call, or address the letter to the proper person. (c) State the reason for the call or the letter. ("Your account is past due.") (d) Be pleasant, but be firm. ("You are generally prompt with your payments; we wondered if this has been overlooked.") (e) Get a commitment. Make it specific. ("May we expect $150 from you by next Monday?") Then mark that commitment in your tickler file and follow up next Monday if there has been no response. (f) End the contact graciously. Do not get pulled into all the financial problems of the client. (g) Be prepared to offer a payment plan that is suitable to both the client and the physician.

10. Have a clearly established practice of when, if ever, to turn the account over to a collection agency, to collect the balance due in small claims court, or to write off the balance as a loss.

Collection Don'ts

The Federal Trade Commission has specific regulations for debt collection. They include the following:

1. Do not misrepresent who you are or why you are contacting a person.
2. Do not send postcards; rather, mail a collection letter.
3. Do not use deception in any form in your contact.
4. Do not telephone at odd hours or make repeated calls or calls to the debtor's friends, relatives, neighbors, employers, or children. Acceptable hours to call are 8 A.M. to 9 P.M.
5. Do not threaten or falsely assert that credit ratings will be hurt.
6. Do not make calls or send letters demanding payment for amounts not owed.
7. If a contact must be made to the debtor's place of business, do not reveal to a third party the reason for the contact. The client's privacy and reputation must be protected.

If your clinic denies credit to a client on the basis of an adverse credit report from a credit bureau or similar agency, you must tell the client the name and address of the agency providing the information, even if you are not asked. Failure to do so could result in legal action. Let clients know that it is their right to obtain a copy of their credit report to see if all the information is correct. A form letter should be available in your clinic that courteously informs the client that credit has been denied; leaving blanks for the name and address of the agency that supplied the credit information. Mail a copy to the client and keep a copy for your records.

Collection Problems

An up-front, matter-of-fact approach to collections will increase the cash flow in the health care setting and make collections easier for everyone. However, every practice has slow payers, hardship cases, skips, and a few who never intend to pay. Move slow payers to a cash basis as soon and as often as possible and yet maintain good public relations.

Hardship cases pose another problem. Anyone might have a time when the payment of a medical bill might be nearly impossible. Care must be taken to be understanding at all times. Try to work out payment plans with the clients so that they, too, are able to take pride in themselves and their ability to pay. Social agencies may be suggested if necessary. If circumstances dictate, providers may choose to write off an account rather than try to collect. That is a decision for the provider.

There will always be a small percentage of clients who never intend to pay their bills. Some of these individuals leave the area, "skipping" out on their financial responsibilities. All possible resources should be exhausted to find the skips and to seek reimbursement. If the client has not skipped but still does not intend to pay, consider taking action in small claims court. Other options are to use a collection agency or to write-off the loss. Providers and physicians often withdraw themselves formally from these cases and encourage the clients to seek treatment elsewhere.

Chapter 4 gives information about the procedures to follow for collecting a bill from the estate of a client who has died. Chapter 4 also provides an explanation of the steps to follow for taking a client to small claims court. Both of these situations are fairly uncomplicated and will produce results worth the effort if employees are consistent and conscientious in these dealings.

Another problem can occur in reimbursement when insurance claims are denied for one reason or another. Successful medical practice management suggests that spending a couple of hours a week appealing denied claims is well worth the effort. Many staff in health care settings lack the time or the skill to be successful in the appeal process. There are service agencies that can be employed to file appeals for denied claims.

▲ CRITICAL THINKING EXERCISE

1. Your employer approaches you and says you are behind in paying your medical bills. He asks if that is true. What collection "don't" has been violated?
2. You are an insurance biller for a large clinic. You delay calling a large family whose members are clients of your practice. You know they will involve you in a complex "hard luck" story that probably is true. Discuss.

Collection Agencies

If you have diligently followed billing and collection procedures and come to the conclusion that the client is not going to pay, you have two options. One option is to write off the account; the other is to turn it over to a collection agency.

Obviously, this decision must be consistent with office policy while still leaving the final decision to the physician or provider who reviews the record. Collection agencies generally are employed as a last resort. Most people, including clients and physicians, tend to have a negative attitude toward collection agencies. However, the agency can be valuable to those who choose to use such professional services.

Selection of an appropriate agency should be made as carefully as one would choose a bank.

1. Does it handle medical and dental accounts exclusively?
2. What methods does it use to collect?
3. What is the agency's financial responsibility?
4. What percentage will the medical practice receive?
5. How promptly does it settle accounts?
6. Does the agency have a good bank reference?

7. How much cost versus goodwill will the practice incur by using this agency?

8. Will it provide you with a list of satisfied customers or references?

9. Will you have the ability to end the agency's collection efforts?

Check with the Better Business Bureau or the local medical association for possible recommendations. An agency that is a member of the American Association of Credit and Collections Professionals will generally adhere to high ethical standards.

Once the agency is selected, all delinquent accounts need to be turned over to it, including any useful nonclinical data. A record should be kept of what has been given to the agency, as well as a running account of the agency's progress. Any contact with the client, whether in person, by phone, or via letter, should cease once the account has been turned over to the collection agency. If the client sends payment to the office, report it immediately to the agency. If clients call regarding the account courteously refer them to the agency.

The collection agency represents the physician or provider and medical staff. Employees should work with the agency to collect the accounts. Consistent high rates of success by an agency in collecting accounts may be a sign that the health care staff lacks sufficient training to be effective in collections.

Reimbursement Attitudes

Reimbursement for physicians and providers in the health care setting is in constant transition. Although a large portion of today's society is covered by some form of health plan, many in managed care, a number of clients are covered by no plan at all. Often these clients will not seek health care or will request detailed information about your physician-employee's billing practices if they do. Payment plans may need to be established. Also, providers serving in any number of managed care plans will find some plans struggling to find a better method of curbing health care costs. There are some physicians, especially in specialty practices, who refuse to participate in any insurance plan for clients and are doing very well financially.

Regardless of the reimbursement plan, financial status has no bearing on the kind of treatment clients should receive. The Medicaid client should receive the same care as the client who pays cash. Physicians and employees need to be careful of their attitudes toward those clients who have difficulty paying their bills, for whatever reason. Actions often speak louder than words, and clients easily perceive their true meanings.

Ethical Implications

Reimbursement and collection issues bring to the fore ethical implications for discussion. Consider the following questions. None has a simple or easy answer.

▲ Is health care a right or privilege?

▲ Should physicians and providers be able to deny care to anyone?

▲ What is the driving force behind increasing costs of medical care?

▲ Who pays for medical insurance and why is it so costly?

▲ What is the role of government in providing health care, if any?

▲ Who controls client health care? The client, the insurance carrier, the primary care provider, or the government?

▲ CRITICAL THINKING EXERCISE

Often, employees in health care believe they have more client contact when performing clinical procedures. After reading and understanding the complexity of this chapter, discuss the importance of client contact when helping clients understand reimbursement.

Summary

Physicians and health care professionals receive payment for their services through numerous means. Clients come with more than 100 different insurance plans to cover their costs. The complexity of reimbursement challenges both the health professional and the client. Education is paramount for the client; however, there also are numerous laws related to reimbursement and collections that health professionals must understand.

QUESTIONS FOR REVIEW

1. Briefly describe the requirements of the Truth in Lending Law.

2. Name the reimbursement and billing laws that pertain to Medicare and Medicaid.

3. How are DRGs and the ICD-10-CM related to reimbursement and billing?

4. What actions can be taken to help clients be responsible for their medical costs?

5. List at least five collection do's and five collection don'ts.

6. Describe four collection problems.

_____

_____

_____

7. What is a collection agency?

_____

_____

_____

CLASSROOM EXERCISES

1. As a newly employed medical office manager, you discover that one of the physicians in the clinic does not follow the written collections policies and is more lenient about clients paying their bills. What problem does this create for you and the other physicians?

2. A provider overhears the receptionist say to a client, "Well, you know, we can take only so many welfare clients." How can the client now be put at ease?

3. Correct the following telephone conversation:

BOOKKEEPER (BK):	"Hi, this is Dr. Erythro's office. Who's this?"
CLIENT (CL):	"This is Laura Phagocyte."
BK:	"You owe us forty-six dollars and twenty cents. Can you pay us ten dollars today?"
CL:	"Yeah, I'll put it in the mail."
BK:	"Will it be check or money order?"
CL:	"Check."
BK:	"Fine, I'll expect it in a few days. Thank you. Good-bye."

4. You are a bookkeeper for a very busy two-physician clinic. Managing client accounts that are covered under a myriad of insurance plans providing differing reimbursement rates is taking an increasing amount of time and energy. The physicians have already determined not to take any more Medicare or Medicaid clients, and are discussing dropping other insurance plans. What are the legal and ethical implications?

5. You have been asked to do the collection calls in your large medical clinic. Although you work in insurance coding and billing, you are not sure you have the skills to do so. This assignment will also include appealing denied insurance claims. What must you do to be prepared and to be successful?

REFERENCE

1. Cascardo, D. (2006). Bank on it: Polished policies maximize reimbursement. *PMA Today*, Jan–Feb, 18–19.

WEB RESOURCES

▲ Appeal Solution. www.appealsolution.com

▲ Credit Report Problems. www.creditreportproblems.com

▲ "In New Health Plan, Patients Pay Their Share – Or Else," by Sarah Rubenstein, 03/13/06. *The Wall Street Journal*. http://aolsvc.news.aol.com/business/article

▲ Malpractice/Litigation News. www.medicalnewstoday.com

▲ "Medical Dispatch Piecework" by Atul Gawande, Medicine's Money Problem, 04/04/05. *The New Yorker Printables*. www.newyorker.com/printables

▲ Medical Group Management Association. www.mgma.com

▲ Medical News Today, Medical Malpractice/Litigation News. www.medicalnewstoday.com

▲ Medicare. www.medicare.gov

▲ "Physicians Practice Pearls," by Elizabeth Woodcock, MBA. www.physicianpractice.com

CHAPTER 10

Employment Practices

To be successful, the first thing to do is fall in love with your work.

Sister Mary Lauretta

LEARNING OBJECTIVES

Upon successful completion of this chapter, you will be able to:

1. Discuss the importance of policy manuals and personnel policies.
2. Explain, in your own words, the importance of correct hiring practices.
3. Recall one source of information on hiring practices beneficial to physicians and providers.
4. List at least four necessary components of personnel policies.
5. Identify the three necessary elements of job descriptions.
6. Discuss office hours, workweek, benefits, and salaries.
7. Explain, in your own words, where and how to locate prospective employees.
8. List eight techniques for effective interviews.
9. Identify five potential discrimination problems to consider when hiring.
10. Describe sexual harassment, the Occupational Safety and Health Act, and the Americans with Disabilities Act as federal mandates.
11. Explain the three parts of the Occupational Safety and Health Act.
12. Discuss the importance of the Americans with Disabilities Act for employer and employee.
13. Outline the Family Medical Leave Act and its use in the medical practice.
14. Recall procedures for selecting the right employee.
15. Recognize steps that encourage employee longevity.

Vignette: Must Amy go?

Amy Porter, RMA, steps into the office of her manager at the Sheraton Medical Center to submit her resignation as the administrative medical assistant. Amy has thoroughly enjoyed all their clients, being responsible for busy telephones, scheduling appointments, and helping clients with their insurance, but she has taken another position in a day-surgery center near the hospital. Jeff Lyon, her manager, is shocked about her decision. Amy has been with them only for 1½ years and he never dreamed she was looking for another position. Jeff asks, "Why would you leave after such a short time?" Amy hesitates a moment, but decides to tell Jeff. "I have been here this long without any kind of evaluation, no increase in salary, and no opportunity for advancement or additional training. I can do nothing more for this position. I need a challenge, and the surgery center provides that for me. I will miss everyone, especially the clients, but it is time for me to go."

Physicians do not function alone in the ambulatory health care setting. Even physicians who are just starting their practice hire an assistant as soon as possible. Selecting appropriate personnel is an important business task. A provider's current employees commonly are influential or directly involved in the process of hiring additional employees. Hiring and preparing employees to function in specific roles are both expensive and time-consuming tasks. It is important to perform the tasks effectively the first time.

 Major areas of consideration and tasks to perform include the following:

1. Create a policy manual.
2. Establish personnel policies.
3. Determine job descriptions for each position.
4. Locate the best employee for the job.
5. Conduct effective interviews.
6. Select candidates to fulfill the practice's needs.
7. Keep employees for the long term.
8. Evaluate employees on a predetermined and regular basis.

Policy Manual

Policy manuals identify the policies of the practice. Topics such as client confidentiality, smoking, substance abuse, workweek and hours, sexual harassment, attendance, discipline, employee safety, insurance reimbursement policies, scope of client services, and hospitals served may be included. This manual sets the tone for the practice. The policies should be updated from time to time to reflect any changes in the office, but they should always be in writing and available to employees. Figure 10–1 gives an example of a policy statement

---

CONFIDENTIALITY AND NON-DISCLOSURE AGREEMENT

I,_____ , do affirm that I will not divulge
_____[Practice Name]____ DATA TO ANY UNAUTHORIZED PERSON FOR ANY
REASON. Neither will I directly use, or allow the use of, ____[Practice Name]____
DATA for any purpose other than that directly associated with my official
assigned duties. I understand that ALL PATIENT INFORMATION, including
financial data, is strictly confidential.

Furthermore, I will not, either by direct action or by counsel, discuss,
recommend, or suggest to any unauthorized person the nature or content of
any_____[Practice Name]_____ information.

Violation of confidentiality is cause for disciplinary action, including
immediate dismissal.

I understand that signing this document does not preclude me from reporting
instances of breach of confidentiality.

Signed _____   Date _____

FIGURE 10–1 Confidentiality and Non-Disclosure Agreement

regarding a Confidentiality and Non-Disclosure Agreement that employees might be asked to sign. Such a document should be reviewed with employees yearly.

Personnel Policies

Personnel policies are established to identify concerns of employees. Without established personnel policies, providers soon lose control of the management of their own practices. Before a person is hired, providers must determine their staff needs, job descriptions, office hours and workweek, benefits and salaries, and how employees will be evaluated. Providers will want to determine if their employees are to be generalists or specialists in their skills, or if a combination of employees would be more effective. It is important, too, to decide if employees will be cross-trained and if so, for what specific positions. Once these personnel policies have been determined, they should be set in writing in the policy manual.

If the office policy manual is not intended to be a contract between the employer and the employee, but simply a guideline, the manual should clearly state that its terms do not constitute a contract.

Job Descriptions

Job descriptions indicate minimum qualifications required, a description of the job to be performed, and to whom the employee is responsible. Written job descriptions are often shared with candidates at the time of interviews.

Job descriptions must be written and are developed for each position when new jobs are created. Other medical practices may be willing to share their job descriptions. Medical assistant educators and professional organizations can also be helpful resources.

The established health care clinic will find its employees to be the best resources when writing job descriptions. Job descriptions are established by having the employees put in writing descriptions of the tasks they perform in a normal workday. This exercise provides the basis for the job descriptions.

When developing a specific job description, education and training requirements must be included. Equally important, job descriptions should also contain specific physical requirements such as seeing (must be able to read reports and use computer), hearing (must be able to hear well enough to communicate with co-workers), standing/walking, climbing, stooping, lifting, pulling, and so forth. Indicate the frequency with which each physical requirement will be used, such as rarely, frequently, or regularly. This will help ensure that the Americans with Disabilities Act (ADA) is followed and that the right employee is hired to do a specific job. (See page 148–149 for further discussion on ADA.)

Office Hours and Workweek

Office hours and the workweek are generally easier to establish than job descriptions. Hours may be determined by the medical specialty, as well as the dictates of the community. The long and often inconsistent hours of a medical practice should be addressed; for example, will every employee stay late, will hours be staggered, and will overtime be compensated? Will the workweek be the same as or longer than office hours? How will a policy be established that provides for the needs of clients and allows all tasks to be performed?

Employees become unhappy when they are told upon hiring that the workweek will be 40 hours and then it turns out to be closer to 50 or 60 hours. Planning for overtime is essential. Being honest with employees is a must. Employees must plan for their out-of-office responsibilities so that they do not interfere with the office practice. Day-care issues and family needs require firm policies on overtime.

Benefits and Salaries

Benefits and salaries are of concern to both employees and employers. Providers will want to pay a salary that is commensurate with the responsibilities of the task to be performed and that reflects the education, training, and experience of the employees. A third consideration can be the prevailing wage of the community.

Benefits to consider include medical, sick leave, vacations, holidays, retirement, and profit-sharing plans. Other incentives may include payment of educational courses, seminars, professional memberships, a uniform allowance, and possibly a gas allowance. An important benefit, especially in the city, may be free parking or bus passes.

The Employment Process

Locating Employees

A valuable resource for health clinics seeking employees is the county medical society. Some medical societies sponsor a medical employment agency. Schools in the community that have accredited education programs for medical assistants, medical secretaries, or other professionals often have names of graduates seeking employment.

Professional national organizations for medical assistants such as the American Association of Medical Assistants and the American Medical Technologists Association may have a local chapter in your community that may be able to provide possible candidates for employment.

Other providers and their employees often know of potential candidates. Employment agencies specializing in medical and dental employment are other sources. Newspaper advertising may also be successful.

In an established medical practice, the initial screening of candidates is often delegated to an office manager or a specific person other than the physician.

Interview Process

With a printed job description and a list of possible candidates, the interview process can begin. The interview is a time to meet with each candidate personally. A job application may or may not have been completed at this point.

After the interview, take the time to make notes that will serve as a reminder later when considering several candidates. It is wise to inform applicants that you will be taking notes during the interview; otherwise, they may be concerned.

 Commonsense techniques to make the interview more effective include the following:

1. Identify the purpose of the interview and describe the position being filled.

IN THE NEWS

The U.S. Labor Department predicts that for 2007, pay raises will stay at 3.7 percent yet health benefit costs are expected to rise 6.7%. The Department's survey of companies found that most are reluctant to give pay raises because of rising costs especially for energy. Rather, companies prefer pay incentives because they have to be re-earned every year.

2. Avoid interruptions during the interview. Do not rush; however, it is prudent to inform the interviewee that you have a set amount of time for the interview.
3. Use effective communication skills and listen carefully to the candidate.
4. Match the candidate to the job. Look at the total qualifications of the candidate. Do not pick a clone similar to yourself. Look for diversity.
5. Observe nonverbal behavior.
6. Ask each candidate the same questions. These may include the following: What are your qualifications? Why are you leaving your present position? When can you begin work? What salary do you expect? What do you expect to be doing in 1 year? In 5 years? Why do you want to work here? Do you foresee any difficulties that may prevent you from doing a good job? What prompted you to become a medical employee? What is your major strength? Your major weakness?
7. Remain objective.
8. Maintain control of the interview.
9. Present possible scenarios requiring a solution to help determine skill level and communication style.
10. End on a positive note, summarize, allow for questions from the candidate, and provide the candidate with a possible date for a decision.

Selecting Employees

After completion of the interview process, make a careful study of all candidates and their responses to questions. If you have not already done so, employment applications should be read, and references should be contacted. This latter task is one that 75% of employers do not do. Yet talking with former employers and individuals named as references is an important part of the decision-making process. Always ask permission from your perspective employee prior to checking references or include a permission request on the job application form.

 Reference Check Questions:

1. Can you share information about this applicant?
2. Our applicant has listed a position with you as _____. Is this correct?
3. Does the applicant work best as a member of a team or alone?
4. Give an example of this applicant's exemplary performance?
5. How does the applicant perform under stress?
6. Would you rehire this person? Why or why not?
7. Would you recommend the applicant for this specific position?
8. Is there anything else we should know about this applicant?

How each candidate will function with other staff members should be considered. If candidates have been asked to perform any skill functions, the tests should be checked for accuracy. Candidates may be asked to do some keyboarding, take a spelling test (medical and nonmedical words), or perform a clinical function. Telephone candidates or ask them to telephone the office at a later time to screen their telephone personalities. The manner in which candidates handle the telephone is important because the client's first contact with the provider's practice is often made via the telephone.

Once a decision is made, all candidates should be informed. This is an often–overlooked courtesy. Establish a probationary period for the new employee; 3 months is usually adequate time to determine whether or not the working relationship is a good one. At the end of this period, either employee or employer should be free to end the employment agreement. Salary paid during the probationary period may be less than that offered for permanent employment.

Employee Evaluations

Evaluation of employees is an ongoing task throughout the individual's employment. Probably the biggest mistake made in health care employment is not making evaluation a formal process. A clearly established and written evaluation policy and form should be developed and carefully explained to employees. A copy of the evaluation policy and form should also be available to employees. At regular intervals during the course of employment, managers should conduct evaluations. New employees should be evaluated at 3 months, thus ending the probationary period. Another evaluation is conducted 6 months later. Thereafter, yearly evaluations on the date of original hire are conducted. If problems surface or an employee is assigned a new major responsibility, evaluations may change and increase in frequency. Strengths and weaknesses should be documented. The evaluation then should become part of the employee's personnel file.

An adequate evaluation enables employees to improve job performance and serves as a tool for employers to discuss salary increases, provides background for any necessary dismissal, and establishes a record for future referral. Samples of employee evaluation forms may be available through the American Medical Association and resources provided by Medical Group Management Association.

Although the evaluation records may assist a manager in determining salary increases, a change in salary is best handled at the end of each year and discussed with each employee. Salary changes and evaluations should be kept separate. However, a wise manager recognizes the value of an excellent employee and will make the salary reimbursement an encouragement for the employee to remain with the practice.

Employee Termination

When evaluating employees, the decision may be made to terminate an employee. Termination is a difficult, unpleasant situation, but steps must be taken to protect the practice and to minimize the stress for the employee who is terminated.

If the evaluation process has been effective, documentation exists in the employee's personnel file detailing the problem behaviors. The file should include dates the problems were discussed with the employee and specific actions discussed for correction of the problems. It is best to have the employee sign the documents to ensure that the employee has been informed and understands the problem areas and what specific actions are required for correction. Such written documentation will be essential should the terminated employee later seek litigation.

The employee's progress or lack of progress should be evident in the personnel file. Termination should take place during the probationary period if possible. Warnings to the employee help ward off surprise when termination is made. During the termination conference, it is best to be brief, to the point, and honest without degrading the employee.

 There are likely three reasons requiring immediate termination of employment: (1) breach of client confidentiality, (2) disregard for client safety, and (3) fraudulent and/or criminal actions.

The policy manual must clearly identify and define these reasons for immediate termination. Also, it may be best to take any termination action late on a Friday afternoon so that disruption is minimized and there is no opportunity to compromise the medical practice.

Managers can learn from the termination experience. Was the job description clear and accurate? Was the probationary period long enough? Was the evaluation process fair, clear, and well documented? How and when were the problem areas communicated to the employee? However unfortunate termination is to both the employee and employer, it is best to use good human relation skills, express empathy, and communicate clearly your expectations to employees.

IN THE NEWS

The Age Discrimination Employment Act allows employers, without fear of a discrimination judgment, to dismiss incompetent employees who are older than 40. Older employees can be judged against their job requirements and qualifications without regard to age. Companies may base personnel decisions solely on the job requirements for a particular position and on the applicant's ability to meet those requirements as well as or better than any other applicant. However, when lawsuits are filed, employers, not employees, have the burden of proof to show evidence that their actions did not constitute discrimination.

When Employees Choose to Leave

There is any number of reasons for employees to leave a practice. They may find a better job, move, have a change in family responsibilities, or retire. An exit interview should be conducted. This is a time to gather specific information about closing the employment relationship. It is also a time for both employer and employee to evaluate the position and identify any potential changes. Some of the questions you might ask the employee who is leaving include: (1) What did you like the best about your job? (2) What did you like least? (3) What would you change about your position? (4) Did you receive the support that you needed to do your job? (5) What would improve the workplace for someone in your position? (6) Did you receive the feedback you needed? (7) Was your supervisor's management style a key to your leaving? (8) Is there anything else you would like to comment on?

Keeping Employees

Keeping employees is as important as selecting them. Salaries that are commensurate with work performance and the qualifications of employees are a must. Salary is not a place to try to cut clinic expense. The old adage "You get what you pay for" is true in employment. Replacing an employee can cost as much as three to four times a monthly salary.

As important to employees as an adequate salary is the assurance that their work is appreciated and is necessary for efficient functioning in the health care setting. "Thank you" and "Well done" are compliments that foster goodwill and motivate employees to greater effectiveness. Finding out what every member of the staff likes to do best and allowing them to do it will enhance employee satisfaction. Good employees merit trust and increased responsibilities. Encourage employees to improve their education and knowledge, and provide incentives for that. If employees are to be corrected or disciplined, never do so in front of other employees or clients. Most will accept tactful criticism well. Few will forget if they are embarrassed before their peers or the clients. Remembering birthdays and employment anniversaries with simple gifts or cards takes little effort but does much for employee morale.

Employees in the health care setting can make or break a medical practice. Take the time and effort to ensure that staff functions as a team to create an atmosphere conducive to good provider–client relationships.

▲ CRITICAL THINKING EXERCISE

The office manager in a busy medical practice faces the following hiring situations:

1. A transcriptionist uses a wheelchair. The physician groans, "Isn't there someone else? Do you realize the accommodations we'll have to make?"

2. A medical assistant who is morbidly obese is interviewed. The receptionist sarcastically comments, "That's a good role model to have in a cardiologist's office."
3. A female comments to the only male employee in the medical practice, "You know, when we first hired you, I was concerned. But you complement our practice more than any other medical assistant we have ever had."

Discuss.

Legal Implications

Individuals involved in the hiring process need to be knowledgeable about state and federal work and employment regulations. The Department of Labor, Wage, and Hour Division will answer questions regarding minimum wages, use of child labor, and length of workday. Your state human rights commission can answer questions on possible discrimination in the interview or hiring process.

The federal law states that an employer of 15 or more people must not discriminate on any form of application for employment. The discrimination includes age, sex, race, creed, marital status, national origin, color, or disabilities (sensory, mental, or physical). State laws may be more strict than federal law. For example, in the state of Washington an employer of eight or more cannot discriminate.

Nothing in either the federal or state discrimination laws is intended to prevent the employer from hiring only the most qualified person. Obviously, to protect this right, a well-written job description is essential.

REMEMBER... Potential discrimination problem areas include the following:

1. *Age.* Any inquiry implies a preference and is prohibited.
2. *Marital status.* No inquiries are permitted.
3. *Race or color.* No inquiry concerning race or color of skin, hair, eyes, and so forth is permitted.
4. *Sex.* No inquiry is permitted.
5. *Disabilities.* No inquiry is permitted if disabilities or health problems are not related to job performance. If the employer needs to take a handicap into account in determining job placement or fitness to perform, an inquiry can be made.

Most laws permit employers to talk about the job, its duties, and its responsibilities but prohibit any questions unrelated to the job. For example, it is not job related to note that the applicant has children, but it is job related to note whether the applicant indicated problems getting to work or working overtime. Managers preparing for an interview bring a structured outline of subjects to cover with all applicants, and will treat the candidates alike in all respects.

Even though the health care setting may not have 15, or even 8, employees, it is best to follow the state and federal requirements, not only for protection but also for ethical reasons and for good public relations.

 Valid reasons for declining applicants include the following:

1. Applicant has health problem that would preclude the safe and efficient performance of the job.
2. Applicant is not fully available for the work schedule of the particular job (observance of religious holidays not included).
3. Applicant has insufficient skills, training, or experience to perform the duties of the particular job.
4. Another applicant is better qualified.[1]

Family and Medical Leave Act

Another law that may affect medical practice is the Family and Medical Leave Act (FMLA) of 1993. The law applies to organizations with 50 or more employees and will most likely be seen in large medical centers and hospitals. The act provides employees up to 12 weeks of job-protected and unpaid leave for family and medical reasons. The reasons include (1) birth and care of a child as well as adoption or care of a foster child; (2) care of immediate family member who is seriously ill; and (3) care of an employee's own serious health condition. Employees have to have been employed at least 12 months and worked at least 1250 hours during the 12 months before the FMLA leave begins.

Sexual Harassment

Sexual harassment may occur on the job. Title VII of the Civil Rights Act of 1964 protects employees from sexual harassment. The Office of Equal Employment Opportunities guidelines make the employer strictly liable for the acts of supervisory employees, as well as for some acts of harassment by co-workers and clients of the company. A written policy on sexual harassment, detailing inappropriate behavior and stating specific steps to be taken to correct an inappropriate situation, should be established.

The traditional form of harassment is the scenario in which sexual favors are implicit and demanded of an employee by a supervisor in exchange for job advancement. This is known in legal terms as *quid pro quo,* which means "this for that." For example, the physician says to an employee, "You know, there's a hefty raise for you if you spend the weekend on my boat." A second, probably more common form of harassment, a hostile work environment, occurs when the work environment interferes with the employee's work performance. The conduct must be severe or pervasive, and may take the form of a series of sexual questions, comments, jokes, or inappropriate touching by co-workers. For example, a male physician's assistant is always making comments in the front office about "my girls," teasing them about PMS, and telling them that they are inferior to men. When the harassment is commonplace and the supervisor or employer does not correct the situation, the employer is liable under Title VII.

Generally, the easiest way to end harassment is to tell the harasser to stop the behavior. This works in some cases. Telling another colleague or threatening the harasser that you will tell another person is the second best tactic. Ignoring the offensive behavior not only does not work, it is illegal not to take corrective action. If the harassment continues, employers must make it easy and safe for those being harassed to seek help and harassment must stop.

REMEMBER... The policy should include at least the following:

1. A statement that sexual harassment of employees and a hostile work environment will not be tolerated.
2. A statement that an employee who feels harassed needs to bring the matter to the immediate attention of a person designated in the policy.
3. A statement about the confidentiality of any incidents and specific disciplinary action against the harasser.
4. The procedure to follow when harassment occurs.

Occupational Safety and Health Act

Congress passed the Occupational Safety and Health Act to prevent workplace disease and injuries. This statute applies to virtually every U.S. employer. The general purpose of the act is to require all employers to ensure employee safety and health.

 The Occupational Safety and Health Administration (OSHA) is authorized to:

1. Encourage employers and employees to reduce workplace hazards and to implement new and improved health programs.

2. Establish "separate but dependent responsibilities and rights" for employers and employees for the achievement of better safety and health conditions.

3. Maintain a record-keeping system to monitor job-related injuries and illnesses.

4. Develop mandatory job safety and health standards and enforce them effectively.

OSHA may make unannounced visits to the workplace and may issue citations or penalties of up to $7000 per violation to an employer who does not provide a safe environment.

Contained in the OSHA regulation is the clinical hygiene plan (CHP) that addresses training, information requirements, and provisions that must be implemented for chemical exposure in the ambulatory health care setting. Chemical inventories must be taken, a material safety data sheet (MSDS) manual has to be assembled, and employers are required to provide a hazard communication education program to employees within 30 days of hire.

 The regulation has two standards: the Occupational Exposure to Hazardous Chemicals Standard and the Bloodborne Pathogen Standard.

The Occupational Exposure to Hazardous Chemicals Standard requires the following tasks to be performed by employers:

1. Inventory any and all hazardous chemicals regarding quantity, manufacturer's name, address, and chemical hazard classification.

2. Assemble MSDSs from manufacturers. The sheets should be kept in a manual and reviewed regularly. Label the chemicals using the National Fire Protection Association's color and number method.

3. Provide educational training to all employees who handle any hazardous chemicals within 30 days of employment and before an employee is allowed to handle the chemicals.

4. Develop and evaluate a chemical hygiene plan to address how to handle any spills or exposures.

 The Bloodborne Pathogen Standard became effective in 1992. Its primary goal is to reduce occupational-related cases of HIV/AIDS and hepatitis B and C infections among health care workers.

The Bloodborne Pathogen Standard addresses the following:

1. Control of and determination of exposure
2. Universal precautions
3. Hepatitis B virus vaccine
4. Postexposure follow-up
5. Labeling and disposal of biologic wastes
6. Housekeeping and laundry functions
7. Employee training for safety and documentation

In 2001, in response to the Needlestick Safety and Prevention Act, OSHA revised the Bloodborne Pathogens Standard. The revised standard clarifies the need for employers to select safer needle devices and to involve employees in identifying and choosing these devices. The updated standard also requires employers to maintain a log of injuries from contaminated sharps.

For the safety of employees and all clients, carefully following and monitoring these regulations is essential. Job descriptions should identify any position that may cause exposure to hazardous chemicals, bloodborne pathogens, and needle sticks.

Americans with Disabilities Act

The Americans with Disabilities Act (ADA) was passed in Congress in 1990 to eliminate discrimination in employment against a qualified individual with a disability. The statute applies to all persons with substantial impairment that significantly

---

IN THE NEWS

In 2006, the CDC reported that "Every year 600,000 to 800,000 occupational needlestick in-juries are estimated to occur and can lead to serious or potentially fatal infections with blood-borne pathogens such as hepatitis B virus, hepatitis C virus, or human immunodeficiency virus (HIV). The precise number of injuries is not known because needlesticks often go unreported. The risk of a bloodborne infection may not be immediately recognized, and symptoms may not become apparent until weeks or months after the needlestick."

---

limits a major function. This includes hearing, seeing, speaking, walking, breathing, per-forming manual tasks, caring for oneself, learning, and working. It also protects persons with a history of cancer in remission, persons with a history of mental illness, and persons with AIDS or who are HIV positive.

If an employee who has a disability meets all of the qualifications of the job, the em-ployer must make "reasonable" accommodation for the disability. The employer is not re-quired to make an accommodation that imposes "undue hardship" or requires an action with significant difficulty or expense.

 Accommodations might include the following:

1. Handicap parking
2. Ramps or elevators
3. Electronic or easily opened doors
4. Hallways with at least 36 inches of clearance
5. Accessible bathroom and lunchroom facilities
6. Reception counters low enough for a wheelchair (34 inches maximum)

For example, if the best qualified applicant for receptionist has permanent and serious fa-cial scarring, the applicant cannot be denied the position simply because of the fear of "neg-ative reactions" from others. A transcriptionist in a wheel chair should be hired if she or he is the best candidate for the job. In all probability, reasonable accommodation can be made for this individual.

The employment provisions of the ADA are enforced under the same policies of discrimi-nation under Title VII. Remedies may include hiring, reinstatement, back pay, and the order to stop discrimination.

Most employers with the foresight to hire persons with disabilities and to make the neces-sary accommodations have found that those employees are among the best.

Summary

Outside of concern for appropriate client care, treatment, and comfort, the most important function of the manager and physician will be hiring employees and keeping them. Legal implications of not having good hiring and employment practices and keeping good employ-ees are far reaching and essential to the process.

State laws and regulations concerning employees must be considered. Some states regu-late medical assistants or require their certification to practice. Some states require a license, a registration, or a certification for certain special or invasive procedures that medical assis-tants perform. In employment practices, the smartest step that can be taken is to hire the best educated and credentialed individuals for the positions. Refer to Chapter 3 for further infor-mation on credentialing and education.

IN THE NEWS

In the United Kingdom, legislation protects employees from discrimination of different types.

1. **Direct discrimination** happens when an employer treats an employee less favorably because of gender, marital status, gender reassignment, pregnancy, sexual orientation, disability, race, color, ethnic background, nationality, religion or belief, age, working part time, or working on a fixed-term contract. An example of direct discrimination is when a driving job is only open to male applicants.
2. **Indirect discrimination** is when a condition that disadvantages one group of people more than another. For example, in hiring saying that applicants for a job must be clean shaven puts members of some religious groups at a disadvantage. Yet if the employer can show that there is a good reason for the condition, there is no discrimination. In the example, the clean shaving might be justified if the job involves handling of food and the employer could show that having a beard or moustache was a genuine hygiene risk.

Compare this discrimination law with the United States' laws.

QUESTIONS FOR REVIEW

1. A job description is essential for the following reasons:

_____

_____

2. List possible benefits to offer a health care employee.

_____

_____

3. Describe the important steps in the employment process.

_____

_____

4. List some potential discrimination problems.

_____

_____

5. Give an example of sexual harassment in the health care setting.

_____

_____

6. Name appropriate action to be taken in a case of sexual harassment.

_____

_____

7. Describe the OSHA standards discussed in the text.

_____

_____

8. The ADA laws apply to the health care setting in the following ways:

_____

_____

CLASSROOM EXERCISES

1. In "Must Amy Go?" what might Jeff Lyon have done differently to ensure that Amy would be a long-term employee? What actions should Jeff now take?

2. When interviewing a candidate, a question is asked that the candidate refuses to answer, citing discrimination as a reason. What should you do?

3. The physician says to the assistant in the hall, "I'm tired of telling you how to do things and having you mess it up during an exam. Pick up your check at the end of the week and don't come back." How could this situation be prevented by using wise employment practices?

4. Under what conditions might clinic hours and an employee's actual workweek be different? Why?

5. Your supervisor makes lewd remarks and obvious sexual advances. What will you do?

6. Dream a little. You have the "perfect" employee and want to show your appreciation. What might you do?

7. As a potential employee, answer the candidate questions listed in number six under "Interview Process."

8. You find the right candidate for the job who is wheelchair dependent. What will you do?

9. For the position of clinical medical assistant, identify standards related to hazardous chemicals, bloodborne pathogens, and needlesticks that must be in place.

REFERENCE

1. Fullner, W: Complying with the State Law Against Discrimination in Employment. Association of Washington Business in cooperation with the Washington State Human Rights Commission, Wash.

WEB RESOURCES

▲ About Human Resources. http://humanresources.about.com
▲ Human Resources: Business and Legal Reports. http://hr.blr.com
▲ NOLO Human Resources and Legal Solutions for Consumers and Small Businesses. www.nolo.com
▲ Patrick H. Gaughan, J.D., MBA, Management Help, LLC. www.managementhelp.org
▲ The Job Stores. www.jobstores.com
▲ U.S. Department of Labor. www.dol.gov

CHAPTER 11

A Cultural Perspective for Health Professionals

> " *As different as we are from one another, as unique as each one of us is, we are much more the same than we are different. That may be the most essential message of all, as we help our children grow toward being caring, compassionate, and charitable adults.* "
>
> *Fred Rogers*

LEARNING OBJECTIVES

Upon successful completion of this chapter, you will be able to:

1. Discuss the impact of cultural influence on health care.
2. Identify the stages of sensitivity to cultural diversity.
3. Recall the components of cultural diversity.
4. Give an example of each component of cultural diversity.
5. Examine the concept of a new culture.
6. Evaluate self as related to cultural sensitivity.
7. Identify any personal prejudice or bias and determine a strategy to address it.
8. Facilitate cross-cultural communication.

Vignette: Who is the healer?

In a Southwestern region of the United States, a Native American healer was called at the same time as an ambulance. Before the ambulance crew could begin their work, the healer performed a "purification" or "healing ritual" on the afflicted person.

In today's society that is increasingly mobile, clients come from all cultural backgrounds seeking health care. Each of us is a member of a particular cultural heritage that is always with us, defines who we are, and includes bias, prejudice, and preconceived notions about others whose culture is different. Sometimes cultural variances are obvious either by color, dress, stature, or action. Sometimes cultural differences are obscure. Health professionals who understand and appreciate their own culture are more able to embrace those from differing cultures.

How do we address cultural differences? Do we understand client's mores that differ from our own? Are we accepting of differences and similarities? Are we open-minded? How will a better understanding of cultures help us be more effective health care practitioners? Cultural differences exist relative to age, gender, sexual orientation, ethnic background, educational preparation, life experiences, spiritual influences, role models and mentors, economics, values, internal milieu, and health and illness. (Fig. 11–1).

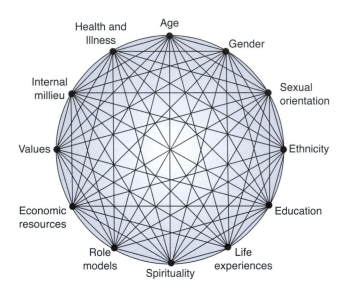

FIGURE 11–1 Be respectful of the differences that make us unique.

Understanding Cultural Diversity

Being aware of cultural differences must be a goal for all health professionals who desire to perform legally, ethically, and therapeutically in their employment environment. Refer to the diagram in Figure 11–2 based on information from Larry D. Purnell and Betty J. Paulanka in their book *Transcultural Health Care.*

In the first stage, individuals are unaware that they lack knowledge of cultural diversity. The second stage, individuals become aware that they lack knowledge of diversity. In the third stage, individuals begin to learn about cultural diversity, verify known generalizations of the culture, and begin to provide culturally sensitive care. In the fourth and last stage, individuals automatically provide culturally sensitive care without thinking about it. These stages are a continuous cycle. To be culturally sensitive implies that you are always learning and growing. Embrace your culture and your stage of development as you progress through this chapter. The goal is to function in the third and fourth stages of cultural sensitivity.

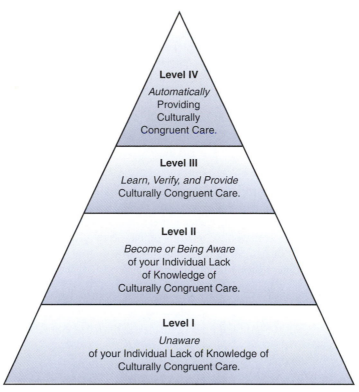

FIGURE 11–2 Cultural Congruent Care Levels.

Components of Cultural Diversity

Ageism is any form of prejudice, bias, or discrimination that negatively targets the person on the basis of age. Children may be seen as property to possess rather than trust to care for and nurture; adolescents may be seen as moody people who seldom listen to others and are diffi-cult to understand. Elders may be seen as hard of hearing, forgetful, opinionated, and set in their ways. The importance of age differs among cultures.

> *The Wang family is elderly. They are Chinese. Mrs. Wang has difficulty walking and has severe kyphosis. Mr. Wang loves his garden, but has circulatory problems. He finds it increasingly difficult to cultivate his vegetables and help his wife. The Wang children are moving their Mother and Father into the home of the eldest son who has already prepared his home for the two of them.*
>
> *Next door to the Wang family is another elderly couple. Mr. and Mrs. Johnson are struggling to stay in their home, but their children are pressing them to enter into an assisted living facility where their meals will be prepared for them and someone will make sure they take their medications. Mr. Johnson worries that he will have to give up his car.*
>
> *How do these examples demonstrate a value for the elderly? Explain.*

Gender issues arise from prejudices, biases, and discrimination based on sexual identity, whether you are a woman or man. It is sometimes used to refer to sex-based categories. For example, in some cultures men may be seen as dominant, athletic, mathematically inclined, and physically superior, whereas women may be seen as intuitive, caregivers, nurturers, and physically weak. Cultures may differ in their views of gender. Medical research in the

United States has been predominantly done on men. More recently, studies are now being done on women. In some cultures, women may take the lead in raising children, whereas in other cultures, the men may. In the United States, some professions are predominantly male; however, that does not prohibit women from entering those fields. In some countries, women would not work out of the home. In other countries, there is no distinction between men and women in the work they perform.

> *Your son plays soccer with a teenager from Iran. In the locker room, Mahyar tells your son about his latest escapade with a teenage girl in his class. He brags that it is cool American girls are so willing when his own sister must still be a virgin when she marries.*
> *What does this tell about the role of young women in different cultures?*

Sexual orientation addresses issues of heterosexuals, gays, lesbians, bisexuals, and transvestites. In the United States, some states address sexual orientation in law. However, widespread discrimination is common. A person's sexual orientation is important to an individual's health care not only in what pathology might be unique to the relationship, but also in the effects of illness on significant others.

> *Gerry and Chuck are a gay couple. They have been together for many years. When the opportunity came for legal same-sex marriage, they tied the knot. Their parents don't think much of this relationship and tell everyone that they are just good friends, but as the legality of same-sex marriages comes under increased scrutiny, Gerry and Chuck are actively involved in their state's legislation.*
> *Is this like your culture? Discuss.*

Ethnic background is one's national heritage, race, tribe, clan, and language and may be related to geographic location. It is estimated that by 2050 Hispanics will be the largest ethnic group in the United States, yet not many U.S. citizens speak Spanish, and many Hispanics speak only a little English. The language barrier often implies that people have not yet learned to "think" in English; rather, they think in their native language and then translate into English. Family plays an important role in most cultures and is key to ethnic identity. Physical space, form of greeting, and eye-to-eye contact vary with cultures. Some professionals are respected more than others in differing cultures.

> *A 15-month-old Puerto Rican child enters the urgent care center with a history of persistent, productive cough, fever, sleeplessness, and congestion. The child is diagnosed with pneumonia and is to be hospitalized. The child is wearing a pretty bracelet with black and red stone beads. The mother explains that this bracelet is what protects the infant from the evil eye. Two hours later, a hospital nurse removes the bracelet.*
> *Discuss the implication.*

Educational preparation is one's formal education, such as kindergarten through high school; some cultures provide children with only 4 or 5 years of formal education. In other cultures, private education is the norm. Such differences may include private, public, or parochial education, even home schooling. People moving to the United States may come with a high level of skill and education recognized in their country but are forced to take low-paying, menial jobs because of language barriers and/or lack of recognition for their level of accomplishment. An example of this is seen when doctors coming from another country must re-educate themselves in the United States prior to taking the licensing examination. Others may come with limited education and are able to reap benefits from the United States education system. For others, language barriers may prevent them from progressing in our education system.

Two expectant mothers come to the women's clinic for their prenatal care. One woman of Appalachian heritage has limited educational preparation. The other woman is a PhD from the nursing department in the local university. Each is having their first child.

  What are the implications for each of these women and/or for the health care professional?

Life experiences include such events as death, divorce, disability, chronic illness, family crises, adoption, and surrogacy. Some people have siblings; others may be an only child; some may have been raised with extended family members. These experiences shape how individuals adjust to life's challenges. Survivors of the Holocaust and survivors of other countries that have experienced ethnic cleansing have seen and experienced persecution that few can comprehend. Such countries include Darfur, Sudan, Bosnia-Herzegovina, Croatia, Kosovo, and Rwanda. Veterans of wars experience events that shape their lives forever. They experience death and destruction few know. Divorce may be impossible in some cultures yet simple to obtain in others. Some cultures view disabilities as shameful, and people with disabilities may be hidden away. Other cultures give a person with disabilities great respect.

Jared was 18 when he went into the military. He wanted nothing more than to serve his country. He had his wish. He spent time in Croatia, Bosnia, and Afghanistan. Few can imagine the violence and devastation that Jared saw and experienced while helping to retrieve bodies from the war zone. He returned home after two terms of service, disillusioned with the entire military experience. He felt his future was in question, and found it difficult to integrate back into society. His former friends were strangers to him. He was diagnosed with post-traumatic stress syndrome.

  How does the health care professional relate to this client?

Spiritual influences may include any of the major religions or no specific religion. A person's belief system may be a separate and unique spiritual support system. Individuals with a belief in a supreme deity may be better prepared for surgery. They tend to "let another take charge." Some individuals are more ready for death and tend to accept it more easily because of their religious beliefs. Sometimes, too, people may view illness or disease as a "punishment" because of their religious views.

Rev. Jesse Morris is a retired clergyman. His faith has been strong for more than 70 years. He has a serious illness that will take his life in a short period of time. His nurse has tears in her eyes as she gives him a shot for pain. Rev. Morris says, "It is okay. I am fine. I am ready. I have a better place to go."

  Is there a place for spirituality in health care? Justify your response.

Role models and mentors may be family members, teachers, famous persons, pacifists, or warriors, and they may have a positive or a negative affect on individuals. Role models and mentors differ within cultures; however, the way in which health care is role modeled is often the way one will use health care. For example, if health care is seen as a right by parents, children often will expect the same or more. If health care is a luxury, however, then it is not expected or sought.

Cherylinn's step brother was addicted to drugs. He had a couple of pit bull dogs who guarded his house while he made meth. His life was a mess, but after his suicide, Cherylinn's Dad took her to see his place. It was both shocking and sad. Cherylinn's response to the experience was, "I will never use drugs as long as I live. I cannot understand why someone could get to such a place."

What kind of statement did Cherylinn's step brother make for her as a role model? What did Cherylinn learn from this visit?

Economic influences stem from resources available, wealth and its distribution, the developing world versus industrial or informational affluence, dictatorship versus democracy. Individuals who do not have the economic resources to pay for their health care may do without. It may be difficult for people who come from a socialist health care system to adjust to a democracy. The third-party payer idea is an economic consideration. Some people may be able to pay cash and receive the care needed, whereas in other countries, it would be impossible to receive such services. In preventive medicine, we require inoculations, whereas in underdeveloped countries, people die from diseases these inoculations can prevent.

A young mother works for a community service agency. She receives little or no child support from her former husband. She has no health insurance other than Medicaid. She has an abscessed tooth. The dentist says she needs a root canal. She has no funds for either the antibiotics to treat the abscess or to have the root canal. The dentist can only pull the tooth.
Why is adequate dental care not accessible to this mother?

Values are morals or standards that are acceptable and practical in a culture. The value of life versus the value of death is a standard set by a culture. Values are determined by culture, family, religious beliefs, school, friends, and mentors. They are shaped by life experiences. Values are difficult to modify.

In some underdeveloped countries, people will advertise to sell a kidney for money to live on. In other countries, people will offer to donate a kidney to someone unknown to them.
What value do you place on your body?

Internal milieu cannot be seen by people, but it affects one's daily life. Many of the influences addressed previously affect one's internal milieu and how one reacts to life. A person can be diabetic with a chronic heart condition or have low self-esteem, but this may not be obvious. A person's internal milieu will affect how he or she approaches health care.

Cultural differences exist. Every standard and influence is culture bound. What is "right" in one culture may be considered "wrong" in another. We feel most comfortable in our own culture working within our own values.

Ron Harrison is a 68-year-old male. He is active; he plays golf, and eats very healthy food. No one knows that he is a walking time bomb with a cholesterol level of 385.
What does this example tell us about assumptions we sometimes make?

The way a person reacts to *health and illness* is an attitude and a perception that encompasses all of the other cultural components identified here. Although some diseases are endemic and specific to ethnic groups, all cultures share the leading causes of death that are still heart disease, cancer, diabetes, and HIV.

IN THE NEWS

The Bill and Melinda Gates Foundation has given $258.3 million in grants to hasten ways to prevent and treat the disease of malaria, which kills 1.2 million people a year; 2,000 African children every day. The amount spent on malaria research is one-quarter the amount spent on the purchase of Viagra in wealthy countries.

Some individuals are intensively private about their health issues; others may broadcast it to anyone who will listen. Some ignore their health challenges. What implications do these three examples have for health professionals?

Rather than accentuate cultural differences, how can we learn to complement them? Our culture is one among many. It has no special status. We need to develop a knowledge base and acceptance for differences in cultural mores and standards.

Establishing a New Culture in Health Care

Every exchange with a client is a cross-cultural one. Each person brings to that exchange a diverse background, experience, education, age, gender, race, ethnic origin, physical ability, religious belief, and sexual orientation. Developing a new culture, if that is what it might be called, where there is mutual respect, acceptance, and an environment conducive to teamwork among clients, physicians, other health care providers, and health care personnel must be the goal. Health care providers must recognize that the failure to accept such diversity among clients or the inability to embrace one's own differences becomes a barrier to provider–client communication and quality health care.

Entering into a new culture of mutual respect, acceptance, and teamwork does not require total agreement with another person's differences; it merely requires acceptance of those persons for who they are and what they believe. One must be nonjudgmental, which means seeing each person with a "clean and open slate," not one that has been tainted by one's own prejudice and bias. For example, we do not have to alter or change our sexual orientation in order to respect and accept someone of a differing sexual orientation. We must be able to see each person as a unique and special human being who has a right to culturally sensitive treatment.

Such a culture demands that each of us become more accepting and inclusive in our interactions with others. It requires that we become informed and knowledgeable of others' cultures. If several clients are Spanish speaking, we can learn Spanish so that at times we may converse in their language or more clearly understand what is being said. Not only is respect gained, but we learn how hard it is to "think" in a second language.

▲ CRITICAL THINKING EXERCISES

To challenge your thinking further, consider the following scenarios:

A male caregiver who is about 6 feet, 3 inches, and 250 pounds brings a 4-year-old boy into the clinic. It appears obvious that the child has been struck several times. While the physician is attending to the child's injuries, the very nervous caregiver paces to the receptionist's desk, leans over, and says, "My God, what have I done? I did not mean to hit him so hard!" Your response might be, "Get out of my face, you SOB; the police will take care of you!" Or it might be, "How could a brute like you hit a child so small?" Or struggling to be therapeutic, remembering that the abuser is also a victim, and trying to accept this person, obviously distraught and upset, as another human being of equal value, you might reply, "As hard as this is for me, you've taken the first step in realizing your mistake. We're treating the boy now. Please just have a seat, try to remain calm, and I'll have the physician speak with you as soon as she's finished." Identify the conflicting values expressed.

A young Navajo woman employed in the medical clinic where you are employed is expecting her first child in a month. The staff is anxious to have a baby shower for her during lunchtime. When you tell the woman of the plans for her, she is embarrassed but tells you she does not want a shower. She explains that in Navajo culture, preparing for the birth is taboo and forbidden. Together you decide it would be fun to have a shower after the baby is born when she can return to the clinic during lunch and everyone would see the baby. Discuss.

A middle-aged man comes out of the examination room and stops to make a follow-up appointment. You notice the tears in his eyes and ask how you can help. He sobs, "Not only must I go home and tell my wife I've been leading a life as a bisexual, I must also tell her I'm positive for HIV." You can respond by saying, "You play with fire, you're going to get burned. I pity your wife." Or, "Personally, I'd never go home. I'd drive my car off a cliff." Or again you can strive to put your prejudices and biases aside and respond, "How difficult this must be for you. I am sorry. Would it help if you asked your wife to talk with us or to make an appointment with the physician? What can I do for you?" Discuss.

Your physician is treating a woman of Chinese ancestry. She is elderly and has been in this country only a few years. She is often temperamental and angers easily. She tells you as she waves the prescription paper in your face, "No make me take this! Dr. Chin's herbs much better—much cheaper, too!" You can say, "You crazy old lady, just go see your Dr. Chin. Don't bother us any more. Insurance won't pay for him anyway!" Recalling your knowledge of the Chinese culture, and the importance of herbal medication, you can say, "You feel like Dr. Chin's herbs really help more? Did you share that with the physician? It may be OK to take both the herbal medicine and the prescription. Let's ask the physician just to be safe. We want you to get well." Discuss.

Evaluating Self

Cultural competence begins with the honest desire to treat everyone with respect regardless of their cultural heritage. This requires an honest assessment of positive and negative assumptions about others. This is not easy, because no one wants to admit that they are culturally ignorant or harbor negative stereotypes and prejudices. Examine each prejudice or bias you hold. On what assumptions is it based? Do those assumptions have any merit? Ask someone whose judgment you value to assist you in this examination. Recall someone with whom you have great differences. Can you foster the kind of respect and acceptance of that person to enable you to see him or her as a human being with equal merit rather than as a person with whom you disagree?

Cross-Cultural Communication

Facilitating cross-cultural communication requires sensitivity to differences, attentive listening, and a respectful, nonjudgmental attitude. However, conflicts will arise. To deal with cultural conflicts pay close attention to body language, language barriers, and tone of voice. The use of a translator who is not a family member may prove to be beneficial. A nonfamily member is less likely to do more than interpret and give advice as well.

REMEMBER... It is the responsibility of health care providers to make certain that an interpreter is available when necessary to ensure the client's full understanding of procedures and treatment.

When negative emotions expressed during a cultural conflict are yours, it is a good idea to step back, breathe deeply, and control your own emotions first. Then ask clients to express their experiences and feelings, if possible, and acknowledge them. Help clients find options suitable to them, and compromise over treatment goals and modalities whenever possible.

Summary

You examined cultural diversity in this chapter and had the opportunity to consider your personal feelings and to recognize the importance of cultural diversity in every client interaction. Continually evaluate your behavior so that your actions reflect an automatic sensitivity to cultural differences. In the next section on bioethical issues, your culture and your belief system will be challenged. In each situation, strive to remain as free of prejudice as possible, thus allowing open examination of all sides of an issue. Consider the following quotes:

> *"The real act of discovery consists not in finding new lands, but in seeing with new eyes." Marcel Proust*
>
> *"A new idea is first condemned as ridiculous and then dismissed as trivial, until finally, it becomes what everybody knows." William James*

QUESTIONS FOR REVIEW

1. Explain the idea of a new culture in health care.

_____

_____

_____

_____

_____

2. List 9 of the 12 components of cultural diversity.

_____

_____

_____

_____

_____

CLASSROOM EXERCISES

1. In each of the scenarios given in the chapter what would be your response? Is your response accepting and nonjudgmental?

2. Interview two persons who are of a different culture than your own. Ask them how they access health care. What is the influence of the family unit? Who makes health care decisions?

3. Recall a time when you personally have been discriminated against in the health care setting because of your culture.

4. What role models and mentors have influenced your choice of health care?

5. Identify the largest ethnic minority in your geographic location. How are the health needs of this group addressed? What do you know about this group's culture?

6. What are the laws in your state addressing discriminatory actions related to sexual orientation?

WEB RESOURCES

▲ The Manager's Electronic Resource Center. http://erc.msh.org

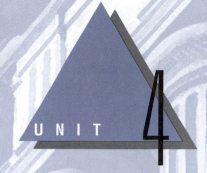

UNIT 4

Bioethical Issues

CHAPTER 12

Allocation of Scarce Medical Resources

> *Due to budget cuts, light at the end of tunnel will be out.*
>
> Bumper sticker on car

KEY TERMS

apgar score System of scoring newborn's physical condition 1 minute and 5 minutes after birth. Heart rate, respiration, muscle tone, response to stimuli, and skin color are measured. Maximum score is 10; those with low scores require immediate attention if they are to survive.

bioethics Morals or ethics connected with biology or medicine.

diagnosis-related groups (DRGs) Categorization of medical services to standardize prospective medical care.

macroallocation System in which distribution decisions are made by large bodies of individuals, usually Congress, health systems agencies, state legislatures, and health insurance companies.

microallocation System in which distribution decisions are made by small groups or individuals, such as hospital staff and physicians.

LEARNING OBJECTIVES

Upon successful completion of this chapter, you will be able to:

1. Define key terms.
2. Explain the phrase *macroallocation of scarce resources.*
3. Describe how decisions are made at the macroallocation level.
4. Explain the phrase *microallocation of scarce resources.*
5. Describe how decisions are made at the microallocation level.
6. Discuss the influence of politics, economics, and ethics on health care.
7. Outline both systems of selection.

Vignette: "Who decides?"

You are employed by a team of transplant surgeons in a major city when a call comes from a hospital that donor organs are available. The wheels move quickly to determine proper matches among the clinic's clients. Your physicians discover that two equally needy clients are waiting for the donor liver. One is an 18-month-old infant whose first liver transplant is being rejected. The other possible recipient is a 7-year-old recently diagnosed with liver failure.

Vignette: Focus on Client

1. A young boy in a rural area of the country dies in a small hospital after an automobile accident. Your physician, on emergency call at the hospital when the ambulance brings in the boy, works feverishly for more than an hour, but the boy dies. Your physician relates to you the next morning the feeling of hopelessness of knowing the boy's life might have been saved if a neurosurgeon and more sophisticated equipment had been accessible to the hospital. Why is it that geographic location may dictate who lives and who dies?

2. The family at 913 Twelfth Street will be saved from financial ruin because Medicare will help defray the costs of their young son's kidney dialysis. The family at 909 Twelfth Street may suffer great financial stress because of increasing medical bills for the treatment of their daughter's juvenile onset diabetes mellitus, which has left her blind and nephrotic. How does our government determine that one medical problem warrants financial assistance and another does not?

3. When a 58-year-old employee, Sam, loses his job because his company is downsizing, he is unable to maintain his health insurance premiums for more than 6 months. He also finds it impossible to find any employment with similar pay and benefits. His wife, receiving care for cancer, is now left without insurance. Sam pays more than $160,000 of his money for his wife's care before her death, just 3 months after the health care coverage was lost. Sam is nearly bankrupt.

Allocation of scarce medical resources and access to medical care are major bioethical concerns in today's society. Allocation refers to the distribution of available health care resources. Access refers to whether people who should have a right to health care are able to receive that care. Winners in this dilemma are healthy and well-insured with good corporate coverage. Losers in this dilemma are often those who are poor, powerless, and persons of color. It is reported that 46 million Americans are living without health insurance. Many more are underinsured.

A large portion of Americans without adequate health care are children. Prenatal care is an unaffordable luxury for the uninsured. Often, adequate care is unavailable even after infants are born. The elderly are increasingly having difficulties obtaining adequate health care. Medicare, with its increasing costs and decreasing coverage, is inadequate. Without a quality Medicare supplement program, the elderly, like the nation's children, will go without. What value do we place on human life in our country when basic health care is not available to those who need it most?

With the ever-changing health care climate and the increased managed care contracts, health professionals in all facets of the industry, ambulatory as well as inpatient care, are required to do more with less. Hospitals and acute care centers have radically altered their delivery system of health care. For example, a surgical nurse with 10 years of experience may be moved to the role of circulating nurse, and a surgical technician with only 9 months of recent training will actually assist the surgeon. The circulating nurse is removed from the actual operation yet is ultimately responsible for the supplies and equipment in the room and documenting any incidents that might occur. Responsibility and accountability issues are shifting toward cost containment. Clients are directly affected, for example, when providers do not take any more Medicare clients and turn away all Medicaid recipients because the providers' costs are not adequately reimbursed.

At the same time, well-insured, and financially successful clients are able to purchase nearly any kind of health care they desire. Expensive nonessential reconstructive surgery, assisted reproduction, and experimental therapies will be made available while the less fortunate are denied access and are given no choice in their health care treatment. The result is there are medical luxuries for a few while others do without.

▲ CRITICAL THINKING EXERCISE

The changes occurring in our nation's health care pose economic, ethical, and political questions:

1. The economic question is "How can scarce resources be allocated in light of the costs required and still satisfy human needs or desires?"
2. The ethical questions are "Is medical care a right or a privilege?" and "How will these scarce resources be justly and fairly distributed?"
3. The political questions are "Who will pay for basic health care?" and "Who decides what kind of benefit package everyone should receive?"

Whenever health care access (providing care for those entitled to it) and allocation (deciding what services should be covered) decisions are made, improving health care should be the primary goal. Health professionals, researchers, and members of nearly all academic disciplines have been formally debating such issues for more years. For discussion, it is easier to define the problem in terms of macroallocation and microallocation of scarce resources.

Macroallocation and Microallocation

Allocation decisions deal with how much shall be expended for medical resources and how these resources are to be distributed (Fig. 12–1).

Macroallocation decisions are made by larger bodies, such as Congress, health systems agencies, state legislatures, health organizations, private foundations, and health insurance companies. For example, Congress determined that Medicare should provide medical care for the client with chronic renal disease. No other chronic disease is specifically named in the Medicare program. Macroallocation decisions also are evident when determinations are made regarding funding of medical research. How much should be allotted for cancer research, for preventive medicine, or for expensive equipment? The health insurance industry largely determines the "reasonable and customary" charges in medical care and therefore what will and will not be covered by health insurance premiums. In addition, Congress has instituted a prospective payment system that reflects macroallocation called **diagnosis-related groups (DRGs),** which categorize clients' conditions and identify them by number. Payment is made on the basis of a predetermined rate or average cost.

Microallocation decisions concerning who shall obtain the resources available are made on an individual basis, usually by local hospital policy and doctors. Decisions at the microallocation level cut deeper into the conscience, because such decisions are personally closer to each of us. Examples requiring these decisions include who is allowed to occupy that one available bed in intensive care? Does the Medicaid client receive the same care as the local VIP? Does a 60-year-old Medicaid client have an equal chance at the kidney transplant as the foreign visitor who has cash to pay for the procedure? Who gets the flu shots when there is not enough vaccine for all those at risk?

The Influence of Politics, Economics, and Ethics on Health Care

States also enter into the political arena of macroallocation. For example, in 1989, Oregon passed the first program for rationing health care in the United States. The Oregon legislature created the Health Services Commission, which, after holding discussions in many public forums, presented a prioritized list of health services they believed warranted diagnosis and treatment. Illnesses below a certain number were not covered either because it was believed the persons would get well on their own or

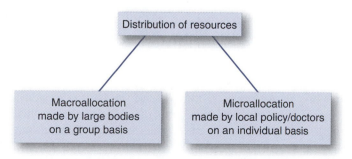

FIGURE 12–1 A brief description of how resources are allocated.

IN THE NEWS

In a business forum on "Health Care Inflation: To Pare Expenses, Ration Services," Robert H. Blank, author of a book on rationing responded to some questions for the *New York Times*. Mr. Blank believes that rationing takes place on three different levels: (1) Macro level where we determine how much we should spend on our nation's health care. (2) Spending priorities. Do we spend the money on preventive and primary care, on curative medicine, or should we emphasize care for the young or the old? (3) Individual priorities. Do we spend it on kidney transplants and if so, how many? Or do we spend it on other procedures? Mr. Blank stated that the United States needs a national commission on rationing to help solve our health care crisis.

treatment would be futile. The Oregon Health Plan extends Medicaid eligibility to all state residents with incomes below the federal poverty level; establishes a high-risk insurance pool for people refused health coverage because of preexisting health conditions; and addresses small businesses by offering them options to provide their employees with the ability to change jobs without losing their health insurance coverage.

In 2006, Massachusetts lawmakers required all its 500,000 uninsured citizens to have some form of health insurance. Every citizen earning $9,500 or less yearly is covered at no cost. Businesses that do not offer health insurance pay a $295 annual fee per employee. Maine passed a law in 2003 to expand health care to its underserved population. Other states with similar actions include Tennessee and Minnesota. Some say such legislation is long overdue; others see such plans as examples of government controlling health care. In any instance, the plans provide for treatable health care coverage, however limited, to all state residents. Only time will address their effectiveness, efficiency, quality, and cost.

▲ CRITICAL THINKING EXERCISE

On a national level in the United States and of worldwide concern is the cost of HIV antiviral drugs. Physicians and pharmaceutical representatives are receiving pressure from persons who have HIV to do something about the antiviral drugs that can cost as much as $20,000 a year. A large portion of the world's AIDS cases are in Africa. How will the nation supply antiviral drugs for its infected individuals?

With advancing medical technology and the increased choices in health care options, we have moved affordable health care outside the reach of many consumers. Employers find it increasingly difficult to include a health care benefits package for employees. Purchasing health care insurance without a group is exorbitant. The American Medical Association (AMA) fought long and hard to prevent government health care reform, fearing the loss of control in decision-making. That control, however, has been compromised by the increasing stipulations of health insurance carriers and managed care contracts. The insurance companies fear they will be responsible for more services than premiums allow. Businesses continue to want to offer good health benefits to attract and to retain employees

---

IN THE NEWS

On a Holistic Health Topics website, it's stated, "Our society is at war. Although it may not be commonly publicized in this manner, make no mistake, our society, and even the world's population in general, is truly at war against a common enemy. That enemy is modern chronic disease." In the United States, we spend 3.5 times more for the chronically ill and disabled than for other health care recipients. The authors' position is that we should spend more on prevention of illness and disease than on the chronically ill.

---

but understand that they cannot pass on those increases to their customers and workers indefinitely.

Whether the issue is macroallocation or microallocation, the problem is how best to maximize the health of the population with available resources.

Systems for Decision-Making

How are the criteria established that attempt to answer such questions of allocation? Two prominent systems have arisen. The first system identifies three possible selection processes. The second system identifies five principles for a fair selection process.

 An outline of the two systems follows:[1]

System I

1. *Combination criteria system.* Those who satisfy the most criteria ought to receive treatment. Such criteria might include the following:
   a. Capacity to benefit from treatment without complications
   b. Ability to contribute financially or experimentally as a research subject
   c. Age and life expectancy
   d. Past and potential future contributions of the client to society
2. *Random selection system.* This system is more like "first come, first served," or a simple chance selection or drawing of lots.
3. *No-treatment system.* This system is based on the premise that if all cannot be treated, treatment should be given to none.

System II

Decisions should be made on the following bases:

1. To everyone an equal share
2. To everyone according to their individual needs
3. To everyone according to their individual efforts
4. To everyone according to their contributions to society
5. To everyone according to their abilities and merits

A summary of the AMA's Council on Ethical and Judicial Affairs suggests that, when making allocation decisions of scarce resources, physicians should only consider ethically appropriate criteria such as quality of life, benefit and duration of benefit, and urgency of need. Such factors as age, ability to pay, patient contribution to illness, or

---

IN THE NEWS

 A *Wall Street Journal* Online July 2006 poll posed the question whether unhealthy individuals should pay more for their health insurance premiums than healthy individuals. (Unhealthy lifestyles were defined as smoking, obesity, and not exercising.) The response showed that 53% said it was fair to require higher premiums. In addition, those surveyed thought it fair to seek higher co-pay and deductibles from the unhealthy. The same poll, however, indicated that respondents do not favor providing a higher level of care for those who make and pay more for their health care. Can you identify which system for decision-making this news report represents? Discuss the ethical implications this poll raises.

---

social worth should not be considered. If the allocation decision poses little disparity among patients who will receive treatment, physicians should use the "first come, first served" approach.

How Would You Decide?

To enable you to appreciate more fully the difficulties in making choices related to the allocation of scarce medical resources and to assist you in establishing a criterion for selection, the following cases are given for you to ponder.

Allocation of Resources
Example 1

On the advice of the staff nurse in an assisted living facility, an 82-year-old woman is transported by Medic 1 to the nearest hospital with suspected fractures after a fall in her bathroom.

Two miles from the hospital, Medic 1 is advised that the hospital emergency room is overflowing and is on divert. Medic 1 continues to the second hospital, 10 additional minutes away. The second hospital emergency area is so busy that two patients on hospital beds are placed in the hallway. After x-rays and a long wait for a physician's examination, it is discovered that there are no fractures, only bruises. The doctor sighs, "I'm so glad to send you back to your home. If you needed hospitalization, I'd have to send you to another hospital an hour's drive away. We do not have one empty bed."

Example 2

*You have just given birth to a 20-oz infant of 6 months' gestation. The **Apgar score** is –2. The infant cannot suck and has no muscle tone, no gag, and no reflux. There is a need to protect the brain and the nervous center. The attending physician approaches you and the infant's father with the news that the only chance of survival is to transport the infant to a neonatal center in the nearest city, 200 miles away from home.*

What is your response? How might the infant's father respond? What problems do you foresee? What are the legal implications of your decision?

After discussing the situation, consider the following circumstances 6 months later. You made the decision to send the infant to the neonatal center. After 2 weeks, your medical bill was well over $300,000. You have only enough money to add to your medical insurance to cover a normal labor and delivery. It appears that the infant will be unable to come home for several weeks, if ever. The infant has now been diagnosed with the following problems: cerebral palsy; blindness; hydrocephalus, which has been alleviated with a shunt in the brain; and seizures.

What choices are available to you and the infant's father now? Who is responsible for the increasing hospital bill? Is medical care a right or a privilege under these circumstances? Who makes the decisions involved in this case?

Example 3

A managed care client calls the medical clinic requesting a different antihistamine because she "has seen an ad on TV" and knows "this medication is the one for me because it causes fewer side effects." You know the medication costs four times as much as the generic, over-the-counter drug she is currently taking. Who decides?

At this point, it should be obvious that no established criteria provide clear-cut solutions to the aforementioned cases. None would be easy to follow. Factors other than those mentioned in the two systems will also influence decisions. They include personal ethics, personal preferences, religion, geographic location, legal requirements, and the political climate. Many problems and few solutions are evident when considering how and to whom scarce medical resources should be allocated.

IN THE NEWS

England has socialized medicine, and some people think the United States should consider such a system. Others believe that we are too culturally different and choice-oriented to even consider it, stating we can't even agree to national health insurance. What do you think? Would England's socialized system make micro- and macroallocation decisions easier?

Allocation of scarce medical resources is a complex issue of **bioethics,** but it is one the health professional cannot ignore because it presents itself frequently.

Summary

Many times allocation and access to scarce medical resources pose more questions than answers. Influences such as economics, geographic location, availability of health care professionals, politics, and insurance coverage determine both allocation and access to health care. How decisions are made and who decides are critical questions to be asked. As a health care provider, it is important to help clients recognize what services are available to them and to help them determine where or how to access other services if needed.

QUESTIONS FOR REVIEW

1. Define and give examples of microallocation and macroallocation.

_____

_____

_____

_____

_____

2. List two influences when making allocation decisions.

_____

_____

_____

_____

_____

3. Describe one system for making an allocation decision in the ambulatory care setting.

_____

_____

_____

_____

_____

CLASSROOM EXERCISES

1. Consider each of the examples at the beginning of the chapter and answer the following questions:
   a. At what level (macroallocation or microallocation) is a decision made?
   b. Can one of the selection systems be applied?

2. On what basis do you decide who gets the last open slot of the physician's appointment book? What system of selection is followed?

3. Two clients desperately need the use of one remaining hemodialysis machine. One is aged and a Medicaid client. The other is a young college student who has full health insurance benefits. Which client would you choose to treat? Support your answer.

4. What suggestions do you have to make health care available to all? How would your plan be funded?

REFERENCE

1. Beauchamp, TL, and Walters, L: Contemporary Issues in Bioethics, ed 4. Wadsworth, Belmont, CA, 1994.

WEB RESOURCES

▲ Strategic Technology Institute. "Toward a Fairer Macroallocation of Biomedical Resources by Constraining Microallocation's Market-Driven Excesses" by Blake L. White. www.ncbi.nlm.nih.gov

CHAPTER 13

Genetic Engineering

> " *In the long run, we shape ourselves, as we shape our lives. And the choices we make are ultimately our own responsibility.* "
>
> *Eleanor Roosevelt*

KEY TERMS

amniocentesis Method of prenatal diagnosis in which a needle is used to withdraw fluid from the amniotic sac within the uterus of a pregnant woman; the fluid withdrawn is tested for genetic anomalies.

artificial insemination Instrumental introduction of semen into the vagina, cervical canal, or uterus so that a woman may conceive.

blastocyst An early embryonic cluster of cells that attaches to the uterus wall and develops into the actual embryo.

chorionic villus sampling (CVS) A method of genetic testing whereby a flexible catheter inserted through the vagina and cervix sucks out a tiny piece of chorionic villi tissue on the outermost layer of the amniotic sac.

Down syndrome Genetic disorder causing a moderate to severe mental retardation. It is marked by a sloping forehead, small ear canals, gray or very light yellow spots at the periphery of the iris, short broad hands with a single palmar crease, a flat nose or absent bridge, low-set ears, and generally dwarfed physique. Also called trisomy 21.

eugenic Improving a species by selective breeding.

heterologous artificial insemination by donor Injection of a donor's semen into the vagina, cervical canal, or uterus to induce conception.

homologous artificial insemination by husband Injection of a husband's semen into the vagina, cervical canal, or uterus to induce conception.

in vitro fertilization Fertilization that takes place in glass dish under laboratory conditions.

phenylketonuria (PKU) Hereditary disease caused by an enzyme deficiency; requires immediately starting a special diet to prevent complications such as mental retardation.

sickle cell anemia Hereditary, chronic form of anemia, affecting principally people of Mediterranean and African ethnic origins.

spina bifida Neural tube defect involving incomplete development of the brain, spinal cord, and/or their protective coverings caused by failure of spine to close properly during development.

surrogate Substitute; someone or something replacing another.

ultrasound Sound waves of extremely high frequency used to examine structures inside the body for diagnostic purposes; produces an image or photograph of an organ or tissue.

LEARNING OBJECTIVES

Upon successful completion of this chapter, you will be able to:

1. Define key terms.
2. List the reasons for genetic testing.
3. Name at least six diseases that can be detected by genetic testing.
4. Compare voluntary and mandatory genetic screening.
5. Describe three tests used for genetic testing.
6. Review the legal and ethical implications of sterilization.
7. Describe the International Human Genome Sequencing Consortium.
8. Describe how gene therapy can be used.
9. Discuss the ethical ramifications between *artificial insemination by husband* (AIH) and *artificial insemination by donor* (AID).
10. Identify circumstances that may warrant AIH and AID.
11. Describe in vitro fertilization and other forms of assisted reproduction.
12. Recall two examples of *surrogacy*.
13. Compare/contrast the following cells: stem, embryonic, adult, and umbilical cord.
14. Identify the use of stem cell research in treating disease.
15. Discuss the use of stem cells in creating "new" organs and tissues.
16. Recall fraudulent claims related to stem cell research.
17. State special considerations for health care employees concerning any area in genetic engineering.

Vignette: "Who has legal authority?"

Parents of a minor and incompetent girl, K.M., petitioned through counsel to be appointed guardians of her person and her estate. They also wanted authorization to consent to her sterilization.

K.M. has an IQ of 40 with a mental age of 6 to 7 years. Her independent functioning is severely limited. K.M.'s neurologist testified that she would never be able to exercise responsible judgment in sexual matters or in caring for a child. K.M. expressed to a counselor that she did not want to have children, but she may have been parroting what she heard her parents say.

The court ruled that K.M. could be sterilized, and her parents were granted authorization. Authorization was withheld pending appeal.

OUTCOME: Reversed and remanded. The court was found in error for not appointing independent counsel for K.M. Juvenile law, case summaries, re the guardianship of K.M., No. 25941-5-1 (Division one), September 16, 1991.

Scientific developments and advances in technology have given rise to moral and social issues of considerable complexity. Recent advancements in genetic engineering, testing, screening, and assisted reproduction enable us to make new choices regarding human procreation and the creation of a healthy society and also raise legal and ethical concerns never before considered.

The federally funded Human Genome Project was completed in 2003 with the actual number of genes encoded still unknown. Studies since the publication of the draft genome sequence have generated widely different estimates. In October 2004, The International Human Genome Sequencing Consortium, led by the United States by the Human Genome Research Institute (NHGRI) and the Department of Energy (DOE), began working on encoding genes. Interestingly enough, it was originally estimated that there were more than 100,000 genes to encode; however, the Consortium has reduced that number to about 20,000 protein-coding genes in the human genome and identified another 2000 DNA segments that are predicted to be protein-coding genes. Human genomes are about 99.9 percent identical; we are far more similar than different.

Not only is gene sequencing allowing us to investigate ways to use genes to prevent or cure disease but certainly allows us to trace where we really come from. More research remains to be done, especially in the use of gene therapy to prevent and treat diseases.

Methods of assisted reproduction are continuing to be developed and refined, allowing people more birth choices. Today many decide to remain childless, seek sterilization, and invest their energies elsewhere. Those who want a child, however, can choose assisted reproduction from a number of different techniques if necessary.

Genetic Screening, Testing, and Counseling

Approximately 4000 genetically related disorders have been identified. In some cases, genetic testing is helpful in treating a client's disorder. In others, no treatment or cure is possible even if genetic testing can detect the carriers of many disorders as well as the sufferers.

Early *voluntary* genetic testing and screening identified persons already suffering from a particular disease. For example, **phenylketonuria (PKU),** a congenital disease resulting in serious neurological deficits in infancy, can be detected when infants are screened within 24 hours of delivery. PKU can be effectively treated with a low protein diet.

Mandatory screening of all newborns for PKU began in 1960, and is now law in most states. Also, some states require that applicants for marriage licenses be tested for the presence of the sickle cell trait, and no states allow the marriage of first cousins; both are examples of genetic screening.

Genetic testing is often used in treating certain lung cancers to determine how well a cancer will respond to a particular drug or drug combination. Genetic tests can inform physicians and pharmacists of how effectively individuals will metabolize certain medications and help to determine a proper dosage. An independent human genome project has been established by a group of volunteers who desire to explore the rewards and risks of making their personal genome sequences a part of a personal health profile.

A DNA sample can be obtained from any tissue, but blood is most often used. Cost of testing can range from hundreds to thousands of dollars, depending on the sizes of the genes and the numbers of mutations tested. Genetic tests are used for several reasons including:

▲ *carrier screening* used to identify unaffected individuals who carry one copy of a gene for a disease requiring two copies for disease expression.

▲ *preimplantation genetic diagnosis* (PGD) used to detect genetic abnormalities prior to in vitro fertilization.
▲ *prenatal diagnostic testing.*
▲ newborn screening.
▲ presymptom testing to predict adult-onset disorders such as Huntington's disease; to estimate the risk of developing adult-onset cancers and Alzheimer's disease.
▲ *confirmation diagnosis* of a particular disease entity.
▲ *forensic/identity testing.*

Pregnant women often choose some form of genetic screening. Typically a sampling of the mother's blood for serum-alpha-fetoprotein testing can detect protein that may indicate **spina bifida,** neural-tube defects, or **Down syndrome**. Ultrasound can identify the size and gestational age and detect some fetal anomalies. For some women at risk, more invasive procedures that gather fetal cells from the amniotic fluid (amniocentesis) or placenta (chorionic villus sampling) are recommended.

Chorionic villus sampling (CVS) is a test used to detect genetic defects as early as the 10th week of pregnancy. In CVS, a flexible catheter inserted through the vagina and cervix sucks out a tiny piece of chorionic villi tissue on the outermost layer of the amniotic sac. This test can detect chromosomal defects. It cannot test for certain brain and spine birth defects, however.

In **amniocentesis,** the physician takes a sample of fluid surrounding the fetus by inserting a sterile needle into the amniotic cavity and withdrawing a small amount of fluid. This fluid, containing fetal cells, is centrifuged to separate the cells from the fluid. The cells are then studied for genetic defects. The procedure is performed no earlier than at 14 weeks of gestation and is generally done between 16 and 18 weeks of gestation.

Ultrasound is used in conjunction with CVS and amniocentesis for placement of the needle. Ultrasound is a fairly common procedure that uses sound waves to produce a reflected image of the fetus on a monitor. Ultrasound also is used to examine structures inside the body, much the same as radiographs but with the advantage that the client is not submitted to harmful radiation. It is used to detect visible birth defects such as spina bifida and heart defects.

The most obvious purpose of such testing is to determine genetic diseases that would cause suffering or death to the offspring, as well as an emotional and/or financial burden on the family. There are two clear indicators to health professionals for the need for amniocentesis. One is advanced maternal age (35 to 40 years of age or older), which greatly increases the risk of Down syndrome. The second is the pregnancy of a woman who has previously borne a child with a genetic disease. The outcome of the procedure also is twofold. One outcome informs prospective parents of the difficulty so they may be better prepared to face the problem at the time of birth and in the future. The second outcome is the practice of selective abortion.

Neither outcome is an easy solution to a genetic disease, especially because the woman already is well into pregnancy by the time the results of amniocentesis are known. Selective abortion at such a stage can be a traumatic experience. All kinds of questions face the client who discovers a genetic disease through prenatal screening amniocentesis: Can I or the child live with the disease, and for how long? How "normal" will our lives be? What financial obligations will this put on the family? How will siblings be affected? Do I have a right to choose an abortion? Does the child have a right to life only or a right to a healthy, normal existence free from pain, agony, and deformity? Who decides? On what basis is a decision made? As technology advances further, a third option might be gene therapy that would include in utero gene replacement or manipulation to correct an abnormality.

IN THE NEWS

Consider the number of world cultures and countries that prefer male offspring to female offspring. Many of these countries have declining female populations, contrary to what is known about population statistics. China traditionally supports the one-child policy as well as the preference for sons. However, due to the change in public opinion the Chinese Government has started a public information pilot project to highlight the status of a female child to recognize her worth and dignity. Chinese law still grants married couples the right to have a single child but allows eligible couples to apply for permission to have a second child if they meet conditions stipulated in local and provincial regulations, which vary widely across the country.

Through gene testing, the sex of the unborn child also can be determined. Although this may serve only as a convenience to parents planning for the birth, geneticists warn that some parents may choose selective abortion on the basis of sex only. Physicians are often reluctant to comply with parental requests to selectively abort a fetus on the basis of sex alone. Recent surveys indicate, however, that only a few couples want to know the sex of their unborn child during the screening process.

Genetic counseling generally is voluntary. Its purpose is to provide information rather than to dictate decisions on reproduction. Its goals are to decrease the number of children suffering from birth defects and genetic diseases and to offer information to prospective parents. However, such counseling can discourage the birth of children carrying harmful genes. When genetic testing becomes part of a medical record, will insurance companies cancel coverage based on test results? Can employees potentially be banned from employment based on test results? Questions exist, such as "Will prenatal testing increase the use of abortions?" "Should any testing be done if no cure exists for the disease?" "Do you really want to know if the news is bad?"

Regulating Genetic Testing

At the present time there are no regulations in the United States to evaluate the accuracy and reliability of genetic testing. Only a few states have established some regulatory guidelines. This lack of guidelines may be particularly troublesome in light of the handful of companies that have started marketing test kits directly to the public. These kits often make claims that they not only test for disease, but also indicate how to tailor medicine, vitamins, and foods to an individual's genetic makeup.

▲ CRITICAL THINKING EXERCISE

To further illustrate the possible effects of genetic testing and screening; consider the following situations and the possible ethical and legal ramifications:

1. A 45-year-old mother of six is expecting. She requests amniocentesis to check for Down syndrome. In an adjacent examination room, a young woman experiencing her first pregnancy is also concerned about Down syndrome. Her sister has the disease. Knowing the tendency can be familial, she also requests amniocentesis. Will the genetic counseling of each woman differ? Support your answer. Each woman asks you, "What would you do in my situation?"

2. Jerry, a 52-year-old physically fit active male faced serious consequences after his second angioplasty and heart bypass. He was again popping nitroglycerin tablets, was nearly incapacitated, and was unable to perform his job as an insurance broker. He seemed to have only one more chance against death; he

decided to take it. Through an experimental procedure, Jerry's heart was injected with a solution containing billions of copies of a gene that triggers blood-vessel growth. Within weeks, Jerry was feeling better. Several weeks later he was working and was nitroglycerin-free. Discuss.

Sterilization

Sterilization is not a new issue. With society's concern about birth control and overpopulation, sterilization has become the most popular form of birth control in the world. Individuals whose genetic testing indicates they are a carrier for serious disease may also consider sterilization.

Sterilization for women is called tubal ligation and involves cutting, tying, cauterizing, or clamping the fallopian tubes so the egg will not meet the sperm and pass into the uterus. Tubal ligations are performed abdominally or vaginally.

Sterilization for men is by vasectomy. The procedure requires a local anesthetic and a small bilateral incision into the scrotum. Each vas deferens is pulled out and ligated. Follow-up of this procedure is important to ensure that all of the sperm have been discharged before sterility occurs. Two consecutive sperm counts must prove negative before any other birth control methods should be discontinued.

Some clients and physicians argue that individuals should have control over their bodies and that they alone should decide whether sterilization should occur. There is a strong argument against sterilization for **eugenic** purposes, and many consider involuntary sterilization mutilation.

States have granted no privilege to spouses or partners for sterilization. Arguments also have been made by the legal guardians of persons with severe mental retardation for eugenic or involuntary sterilization. Refer to the Vignette at the beginning of the chapter.

Another ethical issue to consider is whether sterilization is a valid method of contraception. Society must bear some burden for the attitudinal pressure against large families. Some countries place severe tax penalties on couples who have more than two children. Many countries are conscious of a severe population explosion. Sterilization is the most popular form of contraception worldwide and has greatly increased in the United States.

As so often is the case, physicians and their clients have to make decisions on sterilization alone, with little assistance from the law or agreed-on ethical standards. Physicians may perform sterilization procedures, for any reason, completely within the mandate of state statutes and only after receiving written, informed consent from the individuals involved. Careful counseling should be given in all cases. Physicians should help clients understand that the procedure removes the possibility of having children. Particular care will be taken in sterilizations of young adults who are unmarried or who have no children.

Human Genome Sequencing Consortium and Gene Therapy

With the International Human Genome Sequencing Consortium, more possibilities exist to change how to prevent and treat potentially harmful genes that put offspring at risk or put people at risk for disease in adult years. When mapping leads to any change or manipulation of the gene identified that causes illness or disease, this is known as gene therapy.

Testing for a gene that causes disease will make it possible to diagnose conditions even before some symptoms appear. Presymptomatic diagnosis opens the door to the possibility of preventing the symptoms from occurring. Such diagnosis makes it possible to identify the inheritance for a condition in a family. A family could now know the risk of recurrence in the offspring and also may be able to have information for any possible preventive measures.

Gene therapy is not without concern, however. If genes are to be replaced in the ovum or sperm, the replacement gene is passed on to the next generation. This can be beneficial or harmful. For example, two copies of the gene for sickle cell trait cause sickle cell disease. If you replace the two sickle cell genes with two normal genes, you also eliminate protection from malaria, which is provided by a single copy of the sickle cell.

With all the potential genetic research promises, ethical and legal dilemmas are raised. Some genetic tests do no more than tell persons that some day they will suffer from a dreadful and progressive disease. Genetic tests may force wrenching decisions to be made by parents who may choose to abort rather than give birth to a child carrying a gene for a lethal disease. Or if genetic testing is done later in life, an individual may not be able to do anything to prevent or treat the disease.

As research progresses in gene mapping, there is the potential to alter specific characteristics and appearance. At this point, technology might move from the genetic engineering for the correction of disease into social engineering for the creation of a "superior" race. Some are so fearful of this possibility that they believe all such genetic research should be ended now. Others believe that the genetic age will create a society that is healthier and can be free of a number of debilitating illnesses.

Another question being debated is the use of patent rights to DNA. In fact, about 20 percent of the human genome is patented by the United States Patent and Trademark Office. The United States Department of Health and Human Services currently holds a gene patent that makes the protein the hepatitis A virus uses to attach to cells. About one half of the genes that affect cancer are patented. A private corporation has patented a gene that plays a key role in early spinal cord development. Governments, private individuals, corporations, and research institutes have rushed to patent particular genes in order to claim ownership for future use and research.

The ethical debate is intense. Ethical questions arise. How can someone "own" my genes? More private corporations have gene patents in the United States than public entities. Whose right is it to own a gene? Who decides? Can laws keep up with gene technology?

Assisted Reproduction

Recent scientific and technologic innovations in assisted reproduction have caused us to rethink the concepts of family, parenthood, and human sexuality. The biological concept of family considers those people who are genetically related to be a family. However, this does not include the broader cultural customs and kinships that define family (Fig. 13–1).

Our societal laws determine the definition of family. We have laws on adoption, artificial insemination, surrogacy, foster placement, custody arrangements, and removal of children from homes where they are neglected or abused. Assisted reproduction raises complex issues such as the right to privacy, the right to make childbearing decisions, the interpretation of existing statutes that may relate to this issue, public policies regarding termination of parental rights, and the role of financial compensation in assisted reproduction. We are continually challenged to accept and embrace a broader view of human sexuality and family.

Assisted reproduction choices strain the family unit, the legal system, the health care team, and our values. Any health care professional, whether in an ambulatory care setting or a hospital, cannot adequately function without knowledge of these concerns and their legal and ethical implications.

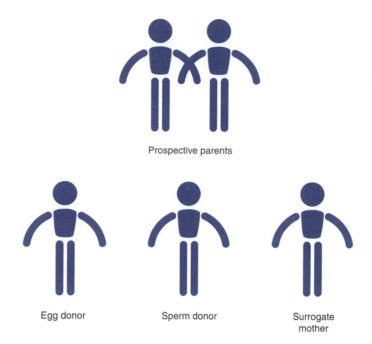

Prospective parents

Egg donor | Sperm donor | Surrogate mother

FIGURE 13–1 Who decides?

Assisted reproduction is a reality. Artificial insemination, in vitro fertilization, and surrogacy have captured popular attention. The use of semen from either a husband or a donor; the fertilization of the ovum in the laboratory for later transplantation in the uterus, fallopian tube, or peritoneum; the use of frozen sperm and embryos; and the services of a surrogate mother provide alternatives to traditional modes of procreation.

IN THE NEWS

Two California physicians were sued by a 33-year-old medical assistant (Benitez) for their refusal to continue fertility treatment for artificial insemination. Benitez had been treated by one of the physicians (Brody) for 11 months who knew she was a lesbian. While Brody was on vacation, Benitez needed a refill of a fertility drug. The second physician in the clinic, Fenton, refused to grant the prescription stating that he and Brody, as well as other employees in the clinic were opposed on religious grounds to treating homosexuals to help them conceive children by artificial insemination. The Benitez suit identified 10 claims against the respondents, including (but not limited to) violation of the California's Unruh Civil Rights Act, breach of contract, negligence, and invasion of privacy. The Respondents replied that Benitez's employee health benefit plan preempted them by ERISA; therefore she had no right to sue. Judgment was ruled in favor of the respondents. The Court of Appeals, however, overruled the respondents. *Benitez v. North Coast Women's Care Medical Group, Inc. et al.*

Can physicians refuse procedures based on religious beliefs? Can treatment be refused to an entire class of individuals? Was a contract breached? What makes the Unruh Civil Rights Act important to this case? How could this entire event have been avoided?

Artificial Insemination

In the United States, as many as 10 percent of couples are unable to have children. For whatever reason, infertility seems to be on the increase. At the same time, the number of infants available for adoption has declined. One possible solution to the dilemma is **artificial insemination.**

Artificial insemination is not a complicated procedure. It is simply the mechanical injection of viable sperm into the vagina, cervical canal, or uterus. This method has been practiced for thousands of years by individuals who had a strong desire to have a child. More than 45,000 children are born by artificial insemination each year.

Artificial insemination is described as (1) **homologous artificial insemination by husband** or (2) **heterologous artificial insemination by donor.** Artificial insemination by husband (AIH) might be used when a husband's sperm vitality is too low or a wife's cervical mucus is too hostile to achieve conception. Semen collected and concentrated over a few days often can overcome a low sperm count or a sperm vitality problem. Artificial insemination by donor (AID) might be used when the partner is sterile or carries serious genetic defects. It has also been used by women who want to have children but who choose not to have sexual intercourse with men.

Obstetricians and gynecologists are asked about AIH and AID almost daily. Physicians in these specialties and their employees need to be able to discuss the topic with intelligence and understanding. Women are sometimes referred by their physician to fertility clinics and specialists which are found in most major cities.

Legal and Ethical Implications of AIH and AID

When a couple decides to proceed with AIH, care must be taken to explain the procedure, its effectiveness, and any possible problems. Permission to perform the procedures should be in writing, with both husband and wife consenting. Confidentiality must be ensured.

Artificial insemination by donor presents problems separate from AIH. Using the semen of a donor other than the woman's husband raises some questions: Does the donor have any right to the child? Should any screening other than for infections and genetic diseases be performed? Can the physician be held liable if careful screening is not adhered to? In the past few years, most states have begun to address these questions legally.

A federal law that has implications for AIH and AID is the 1973 Uniform Parentage Act (UPA). The 2000 and 2002 amendments of the Uniform Parentage Act modernize the law for determining the legal parents of children, and facilitate modern methods of testing for parentage. Parentage determinations must be improved for the enforcement of child support as well. Delaware, Texas, Wyoming, and Washington have adopted versions of the UPA. For example, the state of Washington requires physicians to certify the signatures of consent, the date of insemination and file the consent with the registrar of vital statistics, where the file is kept confidential and sealed similarly to adoption records. Such a procedure or a similar one seems wise when considering the ramifications of records kept only by the physicians involved.

Before performing AIH or AID, physicians need to be aware of the UPA and their state's laws. States with no laws on the subject rely on physicians to act with reasonable care and to protect themselves and their clients in the process. Persons seeking AID are wise to seek legal counsel regarding the legal protection and parentage of the offspring.

For married couples, counseling likely is done to ascertain that both the individuals want AID; however, women have received AID without spousal/partner consent.

A single woman may seek and consent to AID. The written consent of the donor is required in all cases. The donor's signature is required to release all claims of paternity.

Some fertility clinics have a number of donors who can be called to bring semen when asked and usually are paid a fee for their services. Sperm banks provide another alternative for suitable sperm. For information on sperm banks, visit www.spermbankdirectory.com.

Physicians and clinics using the services of sperm donors must screen them carefully and meticulously. Some considerations include a complete physical and psychological examination, a sperm analysis, a genetic history, and appropriate blood tests, including the test for the acquired immunodeficiency syndrome (AIDS) virus. Some physicians prefer donors who have already fathered healthy children. Careful consideration may be given to selecting a donor who has physical characteristics similar to those of the husband or those desired by the woman.

Using frozen sperm for insemination is practiced more commonly. During a 6-month quarantine, the sperm undergoes extensive testing for disorders and diseases, showing a negative result for testing three times every 2 months.

Some physicians who perform AID recommend that the woman seek another physician, if she becomes pregnant, for prenatal care and delivery. This precaution may prevent any unnecessary questions regarding paternity of the newborn and may be wise in states that have not addressed the issue.

Some ethical questions should be considered in the whole realm of artificial insemination. Does the concept of sexuality being tied to the ability to procreate have validity? In other words, some people believe they lose their sexuality if they are unable to procreate. Society places much emphasis on fertility, even though there are many adoptable children in need of loving parents. These children often are not infants, may be multiracial, and may have physical or psychological difficulties. Would society's emphasis be better placed on the needs of such children?

Should artificial insemination be performed on married women only? Who should be a mother? According to some religions, AID is adultery. Is the child then illegitimate?

What occurs in states where no regulations have been enacted? Who monitors physicians practicing AID? Who ensures that donors have been carefully screened? What becomes of the AID records after the death of physicians or when their practices close? Who has the ethical responsibility to prevent the potential marriages of people who have the same father through AID?

Professionals involved in artificial insemination ought to remember that both men and women may be uncomfortable with the knowledge that several members of the medical staff know of their fertility problems and that AIH or AID is being attempted. Health care professionals may have to ask men to manually produce their semen and to explain to women how that semen will be deposited, usually on more than one occasion, in their cervix. Treating these individuals in a professional manner, especially with the recognition that this is not an occasion for slapstick humor, will alleviate clients' anxieties and encourage open communication.

REMEMBER… Artificial insemination is a truly private decision and an extremely personal procedure. Tact and courtesy are essential at all times, and the confidentiality and privacy of those involved must be carefully protected.

In Vitro Fertilization and Other Forms of Assisted Reproduction

The development in genetics of **in vitro fertilization IVF** (literally, "fertilization in glass") is the process of fertilizing the ovum in a culture dish, allowing it to grow, and then implanting it in the uterus. This procedure has been accomplished successfully in several species of animals for many years, and animal breeders have been selectively altering their stock for a better breed. Successful in vitro fertilization and embryo transfer in humans were achieved in the early 1980s.

A benefit of in vitro fertilization is that it allows many women who are infertile because of blocked fallopian tubes or oviducts to bear children. This is done by removing the ovum from the potential mother and placing it in a dish containing blood serum and nutrients. Sperm is added. Once an egg is fertilized, it is then transferred to another dish where, for the next 3 to 6 days, it divides, creating a cluster of cells called a **blastocyst.** The blastocyst is placed in the uterus, where it attaches to the wall and development proceeds.

A number of options are available today to assist with IVF. A woman can have a donor's egg fertilized by her husband's sperm and then implanted into her uterus. A woman can carry an embryo made of a donor's egg and fertilized by a donor's sperm. A woman can receive donated embryos from successfully completed in vitro fertilization. This is sometimes called embryo adoption.

A test that screens for genetic flaws among embryos fertilized through IVF is called preimplantation genetic diagnosis (PGD). With PGD, DNA samples from embryos are analyzed for gene abnormalities that can cause disorders. These results can be used by fertility specialists to select only mutation-free embryos for implantation into the mother's uterus. Only a few specialized centers offer PGD. Prior to PGD, the only options individuals had to determine if there were fetal abnormalities was to undergo CVS in the first trimester or amniocentesis in the second trimester. If abnormalities were found in either trimester, individuals had to determine whether or not to terminate the pregnancy.

Surrogacy

If a woman's eggs and uterus are not functioning, a male's sperm can be injected into another woman **(surrogate)** to fertilize her eggs. This "surrogate," who supplied the eggs, carries the baby. When a woman's eggs are retrieved, inseminated by her partner's sperm, and then transferred to the uterus of another woman, that woman is considered to be a gestational surrogate. Donor eggs and donor sperm can be used to create an embryo placed in the uterus of a gestational surrogate. None of these individuals is genetically related to the child, and an adoption procedure is recommended for legal parentage.

Legal and Ethical Implications of Assisted Reproduction

Informed consent from all involved parties is extremely important in assisted reproduction. The primary role of the physician is to inform clients of all aspects of the process. Clients should be allowed to make all necessary decisions, and

---

IN THE NEWS

Oregon and California are the only two states to allow payment to surrogate mothers for their services. Surrogates may earn $20,000 to $30,000 for surrogacy, while the process itself may cost as much as $100,000. Surrogacy payment has encouraged more women to serve as surrogates because few women are willing to volunteer 9 months of pregnancy when they have no claim on the child. California has become a global center for surrogacy. Oregon also attracts a number of surrogacy clients. Individuals come to California and Oregon from Canada, Australia, and states where compensation for surrogacy is illegal.

physicians should only be facilitators of the process rather than the decision makers. All agreements should be in writing. The physician should certify the signatures of all involved.

Confidentiality is the second legal implication. Physicians and their employees must keep information in the strictest confidence at all times. Discussing such an issue freely, even with the physician, is often difficult for clients. The possibility that any information might become available to a third party through an overheard telephone conversation or a mislaid medical record is intolerable to both the medical profession and the clients. Care must be taken to preserve the dignity of all involved. Comments made by staff need to be pertinent, informative, helpful, and nonjudgmental.

Additional specific concerns, more ethical in nature, must be considered. All forms of assisted reproduction are expensive. Fees can range from $10,000 to $50,000 depending on the procedure. These procedures are most likely not covered by insurance and thus usually performed only for the affluent. Should these procedures be available to all people whether or not they can afford it?

Many argue that assisted reproduction is unnatural and an attempt to "play God." Who are the legal parents of an infant born of assisted reproduction? Perhaps equally critical, what rights does the conceptus have? Are we practicing selective human breeding? Who makes these decisions?

▲ CRITICAL THINKING EXERCISE

A major fertility clinic has a problem. They have a number of frozen embryos stored beyond the recommended 3-year deadline. When the clinic attempted to contact the owners of the embryos, 15 percent could not be found. Should the frozen embryos be donated, destroyed, or given for stem cell research? Who makes these decisions?

Historically, surrogacy received national attention in 1987 when a surrogate mother in Newark, New Jersey, chose not to relinquish the infant she bore to the child's biological father and his wife, who had contracted with the surrogate *(Stern v Whitehead)*. The courts ruled in favor of the biological father and allowed his wife to adopt the infant. The decision was appealed to the New Jersey Supreme Court. In what became known as the "Baby M" case, the New Jersey Supreme Court ruled that the child's father, William Stern, could retain custody of the 22-month-old child but that Mary Beth Whitehead-Grould, the surrogate, maintained her rights as a parent.

In California, Crispina and Mark Calvert hired Anna Johnson to gestate an embryo composed of the Calverts' egg and sperm. The Calverts paid Johnson $10,000 and purchased life insurance for her during pregnancy. During the pregnancy, the Calvert–Johnson relationship soured, and Johnson requested her money earlier than agreed on. Before the delivery of the baby, both the Calverts and Johnson brought suits, each side claiming parental rights. The Orange County Superior Court said that a "three-parent, two-natural mom situation" would confuse the child and "invites financial and emotional extortion." The court concluded that Johnson and "the child are genetic hereditary strangers." The judge compared the contract between the Calverts and Johnson to a common foster-care arrangement in that Johnson was "providing care, protection, and nurture during the period of time that the natural mother, Crispina Calvert, was unable to care for the child."

Obviously, the difficulty in surrogacy arises when the surrogate mother has to relinquish rights to the infant she bore. Some argue that it is similar to baby buying and baby selling. Others argue that without fees surrogate mothers would have little or no reason to offer their services. The New Jersey Supreme Court in the "Baby M" case stated that "baby selling potentially results in the exploitation of all parties involved" and that payment in a surrogacy contract is "illegal and perhaps criminal." Funds do exchange hands, however, and can include such items as $500 maternity clothing allowance; a $100,000 term life insurance policy; $100 daily allowance for lost wages, child care and meals; and attorney fees for the surrogate of $300 to $500.

Finally, any time there is a contract; mistrust on the part of one or more parties is a possibility. Significant legal issues include whether contractual arrangements between the parties are legally enforceable and what parental rights, if any, the participants have in the child. Some states with legislation on the issue have declared surrogacy contracts invalid. Other states have no statutes.

Complex questions are asked: What is the meaning of family? Will lineage be disrupted? What if the parents are unfit? Which relationship takes precedence—that of the adoptive mother and child or that of the surrogate mother and child? Are there any problems that might arise for children born to single women when no father is present? What happens if the infant is deformed? Who makes these decisions?

As long as technology advances further and faster than the legal system can address, these developments and ethical dilemmas will continue.

Definitions of Terms on Cell Tissues
The following terms are defined here to explain some technical concepts.

▲ **Stem cells** are single cells that can regenerate and turn themselves into several types of specialized cells. They come from adult tissues, embryonic cells, and umbilical cord blood.
▲ **Embryonic cells** are cells that are unspecialized that may turn themselves into any type of tissue. They come from frozen in vitro fertilization embryos.
▲ **Adult cells** are those that are found in many kinds of tissue such as bone marrow, skin, and liver.
▲ **Umbilical cord cells** come from the cord blood, and they may contain other types of stem cells.

Of all these cells, the embryonic cells are the most versatile and the most controversial.

Fetal Tissue Research
As early as the 1950s, scientists knew that fetal tissue cells held promise for medical research and advancements in the treatment of numerous diseases and medical conditions including, but not limited to, Parkinson's disease, Alzheimer's disease, Huntington's disease, spinal cord injury, diabetes, and multiple sclerosis. Fetal bone marrow is more effective for transplantation than adult marrow or umbilical cord blood. Fetal retinal transplants are being tested for treatment of macular degeneration.

Fetal tissue research, however, has had a rocky road. Federal funding for such research was severely restricted from the late-1980s to 1993. In 1993, President William Clinton issued an executive order lifting the ban on federal funding for research involving fetal tissue cells, especially those coming from induced abortions. The action was reversed, however, in 2001 when President George W. Bush said there will be no federal funding for stem cell research except for present existing cell lines. There is to be no destruction of embryos (even spare embryos now frozen and some abandoned that are destined for disposal) used for stem cell research or human cloning.

President Bush took additional action in December 2005, in creating a new federal program to collect and store cord blood and expand the current bone marrow registry program to also include cord blood. The Act is known as the Stem Cell Therapeutic and Research Act

IN THE NEWS

China, Japan, South Korea, Singapore, Israel, and the United Kingdom receive generous government support for fetal tissue research and have less political controversy than the United States. There is a trend toward private funding for research. The University of California at San Francisco and Stanford University have received substantial grants. In addition, millions of dollars have come from the Howard Hughes Medical Institute, the Juvenile Diabetes Foundation, and the Michael J. Fox Foundation. A few states have endorsed stem cell studies, also. These states are California, New Jersey, and Connecticut.

of 2005. There is the hope that cord blood cells may be able to differentiate into other cell types in the same way as embryonic stem cells, but without the ethical concerns raised by the intentional destruction of human embryos.

Cord Blood and Stem Cell Research

Stem cells from a single placenta are enough to restore the blood and immune system of a child with leukemia. The stem cells in cord blood can help restore red blood cells in people with **sickle cell anemia.** Human cord blood contains as many stem cells as bone marrow does and is much easier and safer to use as a transplant. Cord blood can be banked and used in the future just as human blood can be.

Tissue and Organ Engineering

Cells can be cultivated from human embryonic stem cells that have the potential one day for allowing researchers to build custom-made organs. If the nation ever moves past the debate on continued research on stem cells to allow therapeutic cloning, it is conceivable that a person with liver failure could be implanted with a "neo-organ" made of liver cells and plastic fibers. Insulin-dependent diabetics may one day forego frequent insulin injections because of a semisynthetic pancreas. Synthetic skin is already available in the United States and has saved many lives. These synthetic tissues for organs are known as neo-organs.

Reproductive Cloning

Many said it would never happen. But it did. In February 1997, the first successful mammalian cloning took place in Scotland when a sheep, "Dolly," was cloned. One week later, Oregon successfully produced genetically identical rhesus monkeys through nuclear transfer. To date, cloning has been successful in cattle, rabbits, horses, deer, mice, goats, and pigs. This is called reproductive cloning. It is interesting to note, however, that the health and longevity of cloned animals is sometimes compromised. "Dolly" died prematurely in 2003 after developing arthritis and cancer, yet she was a mother to six lambs bred the old-fashioned way.

In 2001, agents of the Food and Drug Administration uncovered a secret lab tied to human cloning in the United States. Officials believe the lab was founded by Claude Vorilhon, who is known as the prophet Rael. Bridgette Boisselier heads the group's cloning effort and says, "Cloning a human being isn't just good science, it is a religious imperative." The investigation was held because Boisselier made statements in spring 2001 that the lab was weeks away from being able to clone a human being. Today this claim remains unproven, and most experts consider it a hoax.

In 2004–2005, South Korean scientist Woo Suk Hwang claimed he had cloned a human embryo through government funding and that he had created the world's first cloned dog, Snuppy, an Afghan hound. Months after Hwang published his works in scientific journals, his research came into question. Major ethical violations occurred. Nine of the eleven stem cell lines were discovered not to be cloned. Additional investigation, however, revealed that Snuppy truly was a genetic replica.

Internationally, cloning is controversial. The General Assembly of the United Nations adopted a measure to prohibit all forms of human cloning in August 2005 even though the vote was not unanimous. The basis for the decision was that human cloning was incompatible with human dignity and the protection of human life.

Legal and Ethical Implications of Tissue Cell Research

It is difficult to identify all the legal and ethical implications of tissue research. There are more questions than answers.

In some cultures and countries, human cloning of any form is forbidden. Other cultures and countries are more eager to step into this arena, always pushing science further into the future. Who monitors fraudulent or false research results? Should there be an international advisory group of scientists and ethicists to help determine how tissue research should move forward? If funding for tissue research comes mostly from private entities, who will claim ownership to the results? Should the political climate and leadership in any country determine whether tissue research moves forward? If tissue research has the potential for curing even one devastating disease, why would we not run as fast as possible toward a successful result? How can ethical guidelines and legal regulations keep abreast of medical technology? One thing is certain; tissue research is both exciting and frightening.

Considerations for Health Professionals

Genetic screening, testing, counseling and therapy, sterilization, and assisted reproduction are delicate topics. Because genetic engineering is continually evolving, it is imperative that health professionals remain knowledgeable and up-to-date on scientific discoveries. For clients to be open and honest about their concerns, all employees involved must demonstrate a professional attitude. Confidentiality must be protected. Informed consent is especially important. Employees' personal views on these matters should be fully explored before seeking employment in a facility that actively participates in any procedure related to genetic engineering or assisted reproduction. Also, those personal views should not be made known to clients during or after the decision-making process.

Summary

Genetic engineering of any kind stimulates a number of legal and ethical issues. Legal guidelines are still limited; both legal and ethical concerns have difficulty keeping up with the medical technology and scientific research. The topics included in this chapter are very personal, intimate, and sensitive in nature. Privacy and confidentiality are imperative. As technology marches on, compassion and care are watch words for health care clients.

QUESTIONS FOR REVIEW

1. List the reasons why genetic testing, screening, and counseling are done.

2. Describe sterilization procedures for women and for men.

3. Discuss the work of the International Human Genome Sequencing Consortium.

4. Define AIH, AID and IVF.

5. Identify the various forms of assisted conception.

6. Discuss the legal and ethical implications of assisted reproduction.

_____

_____

_____

_____

_____

7. Describe how cord blood and stem cell research might be useful in health care.

_____

_____

_____

_____

_____

8. Give examples of reproductive cloning.

_____

_____

_____

_____

_____

CLASSROOM EXERCISES

1. Should genetic screening or testing be mandatory for any disease? Support your answer.

2. Sperm bank donors relied on anonymity when they donated their sperm years ago. With new DNA technology, it is possible to trace ancestry including sperm donors. How will the courts respond when a child has a genetic health risk or disease and needs to know about his or her genetic medical history? Will the courts respond as they did with adoption? If a man donated sperm on numerous occasions, what are the implications? Discuss.

3. Should permission of a spouse or partner be mandatory for sterilization or artificial insemination? Explain and justify your response.

4. The California Council of Churches supports a $3 billion state program involving the harvesting of stem cells from destroyed cloned embryos. The Roman Catholic Church says that once a sperm and egg unite, there can never be destruction of embryos. Can these conflicting views be united? Justify your response.

5. A 35-year-old woman comes to the fertility clinic for AID. Her husband is a career naval officer serving on the coast of an Arab country. When the fertility specialist asks about her husband's wishes in this matter, she responds, "Well, we have always wanted a child and it just hasn't happened. I don't want to wait any longer." Discuss the legal and ethical implications of this request.

6. A couple comes into a fertility clinic for AID. They have determined that the husband's brother should be the donor and already have made arrangements with him. What counseling would you suggest?

7. Professor Joseph Fletcher, bioethicist and noted author, says, "It is unethical and morally wrong to deliberately or knowingly bring a diseased child into the world, or to turn a cold shoulder on prenatal tests. Never bring a baby into the world with anything more than minimally serious defects or disease." Discuss.

8. Paul Ramsey, professor of religion at Princeton University, says, "We cannot begin by bloodying ourselves with the killing of our own kind because they are defective in the womb, without also going into infanticide of similarly defective born infants." Discuss.

9. Katherine is a surrogate mother for a couple living 15 miles away. Katherine, near term of pregnancy, decides she does not want to relinquish the baby. What she does not know is that the prospective mother was killed in an auto accident 2 weeks ago. Who has the right to the child? How is a decision made?

10. In the January-February 2006 Hastings Center Report, Mark Greene states, "I propose that serious consideration be given to finding *additional* funding for the purpose of banking stem cell lines that target the African American community. This is not a reallocation of resources within the bank, but a call for supplementary resources." (Vol. 36, No. 1, pp. 57–63, "To Restore Faith and Trust: Justice and Biological Access to Cellular Therapies."). Discuss.

WEB RESOURCES

- ▲ American Society of Reproductive Medicine. www.asrm.org
- ▲ General Assembly of the United Nations. www.un.org
- ▲ March of Dimes. www.marchofdimes.com
- ▲ NARAL Pro-Choice America (Formerly known as the National Abortion & Reproduction League). www.prochooiceamerica.org
- ▲ The White House. www.whitehouse.gov

CHAPTER 14

Abortion

> " *I have met brave women who are exploring the outer edge of human possibility, with no history to guide them, and with a courage to make themselves vulnerable that I find moving beyond words.* "
>
> *Gloria Steinem*

KEY TERMS

conceptus General term referring to any product of conception.

infanticide A type of homicide consisting of killing the newborn.

mitosis The process by which the cell splits into two new cells, each having the same number of chromosomes as the parent cell.

ovum The female germ cell.

quickening The first perceptible movement of the fetus in the uterus.

spermatozoon The male germ cell.

therapeutic abortion Abortion performed to preserve the life or health of the mother.

zygote The fertilized ovum; the cell produced by the union of gametes.

LEARNING OBJECTIVES

Upon successful completion of this chapter, you will be able to:

1. Define key terms.
2. Discuss the use of the terms *abortion* and *miscarriage*.
3. Describe the process of fetal development.
4. List five theories of when life begins.
5. Explain the methods of abortion.

6. Discuss the Supreme Court decisions on abortion from 1973 to the present.
7. Analyze three major ethical issues on abortion.
8. Identify guidelines for abortion in the health care setting.

Vignette: *Where is she today?*

She realized today was her birthday. She wondered what she would be doing. Would she have a party? Would she be traveling? Was she happy and in love with life? Was she as beautiful as she pictured in her mind? Tears filled her eyes. It was difficult to realize that she was not a part of her special day. It was more difficult to realize that when she was born 15 years ago, she could not have been the mother she wanted to be. The decision to give her child up for adoption had been devastating, but even today; she knew it had been right.

Abortion, the termination of pregnancy before the fetus is viable, is a highly emotional issue that elicits controversy no matter what the setting. Medically, the terms *abortion* and *miscarriage* both refer to the termination of pregnancy before the fetus is capable of survival outside the uterus.

Fetal Development

Fertilization occurs when a **spermatozoon** (sperm cell) unites with an **ovum** (egg). Normally, this takes place in the fallopian tubes, after which the fertilized ovum, now called a **zygote,** begins its journey to the uterus (womb). The zygote begins a process of **mitosis** (cell division) during the approximately 3-day journey to the uterus. Mitosis continues while the zygote floats freely in the uterus and begins to attach itself to the uterine lining. The proper term for this attached ball of cells is a *blastocyst.*

The blastocyst continues development and attachment to the uterus until firmly implanted at the end of the second week. From the third week until the end of the eighth week, the blastocyst is called an *embryo.* During this time, organ systems begin to develop, and some features take on a human shape.

At approximately the eighth week, the embryo becomes known as a fetus and is marked by the beginning of brain activity. The term *fetus* is used until the time of birth, usually 9 months after fertilization. The 9-month period is generally divided into three segments, or trimesters. The first trimester is from fertilization to 3 months; the second trimester is from 3 to 6 months into the pregnancy; and the third trimester is from 6 to 9 months (Table 14–1).

When Does Life Begin?

Most definitions of abortion refer to the viability of a fetus. *Viability* means capacity for living and generally refers to a fetus that has reached a certain gestational age and weight and is capable of living outside the uterus. In past years it meant 24 gestational weeks or greater than 500 grams. Although not all agree, some sources now put the time of viability at from 20 to 35 weeks.

 Five possible considerations of when life begins are:

1. at the time of conception.
2. when the brain begins to function, usually at 8 to 12 weeks.
3. at the time of **quickening,** 16 to 18 weeks.
4. at the time of viability, from 20 to 35 weeks.
5. at the time of birth (Fig. 14–1).

Increasingly, however, fetuses delivered before 20 to 22 weeks have survived. Medical technology has made tremendous advances in keeping premature infants alive, making it increasingly difficult to legally define viability. In developing countries, however, where there is little medical technology, the time of viability may surpass 35 weeks.

Some religious groups, including Roman Catholics, claim that life begins at conception because the blastocyst carries the genetic code for a new human being. The theory also is seen in the Chinese and Korean cultures, which count a child as 9 months or 1 year old at the time of birth.

Another determination for the beginning of life is at the time the brain begins to function. Proponents of this theory believe the fetus cannot be a human without a functioning brain.

T A B L E   14.1   **Fetal Development**

End of Week	Size and Weight	Representative Changes
4	³/₁₆ in	Eyes, nose, and ears not yet visible. Backbone and vertebral canal form. Small buds that will develop into arms and legs form. Heart forms and starts beating.
8	1¼ in ¹/₃₀ oz	Ossification begins. Limbs become distinct as arms and legs. Digits are well formed. Major blood vessels form.
12	3 in 1 oz	Eyes almost fully developed but eyelids still fused; external ears present. Appendages are fully formed. Heartbeat can be detected. Body systems continue to develop.
16	6½–7 in 4 oz	Head large in proportion to rest of body. Face takes on human features, and hair appears on head. Many bones ossified and joints begin to form.
20	10–12 in ½–1 lb	Head less disproportionate to rest of body. Fine hair covers body. Rapid development of body systems.
24	11–14 in 1¼–1½ lb	Head becomes even less disproportionate to rest of body. Fine hair covers body. Rapid development of body systems.
28	13–17 in 2½–3 lb	Head and body more proportionate. Skin wrinkled and pink.
32	16½–18 in 4½–5 lb	Testes descend into scrotum. Bones of head are soft.
36	20 in 7–7½ lb	Additional subcutaneous fat accumulates. Nails extend to tips of fingers.

Because there is strong support for the idea that death occurs when the brain ceases to function, it may be logical to believe that life occurs when the brain begins to function.

Quickening has been determined by some to be the beginning of life. Aristotle believed that before quickening, the human fetus had only a vegetable or animal soul. Another reason for this position perhaps is that women truly feel "life" at the time of quickening.

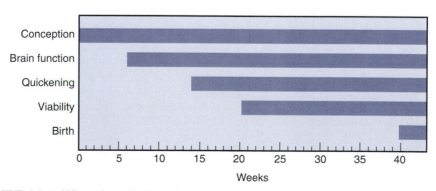

FIGURE 14–1 When does life begin?

The idea that life begins when the fetus is viable or can live independently of the uterus is partly based on the premise that if the fetus indeed can live on its own, life has begun. More variation of time is allowed in this theory if you consider that viability may be sometime between 20 and 35 weeks.

Those who believe that life begins only at the time of actual birth believe so because now the being can be seen, can be held, and is perceived as being fully human. Interestingly, the law states that because viability varies so much, each abortion case needs to be considered on its own.

Vignette: Focus on Client

A married couple has five healthy daughters but want a son. The wife is pregnant and wants prenatal diagnosis solely to learn the sex of the fetus. If the diagnosis cannot be made, the wife wants to abort the fetus. Also, if the diagnosis shows the fetus to be female, she wants to abort the fetus. The husband believes that prenatal diagnosis to determine sex is wrong and does not want to consent to the testing. He convinces his wife to abort the fetus without knowing the sex. An abortion was performed, but the wife agonizes and wonders years later if she made the "right" decision. NOTE: THIS VIGNETTE WAS DERIVED FROM SEVERAL CASE STUDIES BY WERTZ, DC, AND FLETCHER, JC: FATAL KNOWLEDGE? PRENATAL DIAGNOSIS AND SEX SELECTION. HASTINGS CENT REP PP 25–26, MAY/JUNE 1989.

Methods of Abortion

The method of abortion will depend to a great extent on the stage of the pregnancy.[1] Both medicinal and surgical methods are presented.

Mifepristone or medication abortion is known as the pregnancy hormone drug and RU486, is available for use now in the United States to induce abortion. When a woman discovers she is pregnant she may take RU486 up to 49 days from her last menstrual period. The pill blocks the production of progesterone. Forty-eight hours later, the woman takes misoprostol, a prostaglandin, which makes the cervix dilate and the uterus contract. Mifepristone may be the preferred treatment because it is noninvasive, has no risk of infection, requires no anesthesia, is less expensive, and offers greater privacy to women. It can be used in the early stages of pregnancy. Mifepristone also shows promise in the treatment of

---

IN THE NEWS

In Lebanon, Pennsylvania, a rape victim went to a hospital emergency room and requested the morning after pill but was denied. The physician stated it was against his Mennonite religion.

In Washington State, some pharmacists refused to fill morning after pill prescriptions saying it is against their personal beliefs. Initially, the Board of Pharmacy ruled that pharmacists could refuse to fill such prescriptions but due to pressure from Washington State Governor Christine Gregorire, some lawmakers, and women's rights organizations, the Board reversed their original decision.

At this writing, nine states have conscience clauses giving pharmacies the right to refuse to dispense emergency contraception if they morally object. In addition, nine states have policies requiring pharmacists to fill all prescriptions, including emergency contraception.

progesterone-dependent breast cancers, meningioma, endometriosis, fibroid tumors, Cushing syndrome, and the human immunodeficiency virus. Some believe the availability of this medication will only increase abortions. Others say that with the decline of abortion providers and possibly the increased use of the pill, the United States could only see a modest increase in abortions. Millions of women around the world have used mifepristone since it first became available in the late 1980s in France.

Another combination medication for pregnant women who want a nonsurgical abortion is methotrexate and misoprostol. Studies show these drugs take longer because the woman typically takes a dose of methotrexate 3 to 7 days later. She then vaginally inserts a dose of misoprostol. Most woman abort within 24 hours in what seems like a heavy menstrual flow. Both medicinal methods are 95 to 98 percent effective.

The safest and quickest approved method of abortion, if a pregnancy test is positive and it is less than 7 weeks from the last menstruation, is called menstrual extraction, or miniabortion. In this procedure, a tube with a suction device is inserted through the cervix into the uterus (dilation is usually unnecessary). Within 1 to 2 minutes, the lining of the uterine wall and the **conceptus** are suctioned out. A woman undergoing this procedure may experience cramping, nausea, and faintness. It is commonly performed in the ambulatory health care setting.

To terminate pregnancy between the 7th and 14th weeks, a physician performs a suction abortion or curettage. The procedure is similar to the miniabortion. The woman may be sedated or a local anesthetic is given, and the cervix is dilated to permit suction and scraping of the uterine lining. Cramping, nausea, and vomiting may follow the procedure. The client can go home approximately 2 hours afterward. These methods of abortion occur in the first trimester up to the end of the 13th week of pregnancy.

A second trimester abortion, at 14 to 24 weeks, is usually a two-step procedure that can take up to 2 days. The cervix is dilated by gradually inserting a larger plastic/metal rod. The rod may be left in overnight, depending on how far along the pregnancy is. Antibiotics and pain medication may be required. A local anesthetic is given to numb the cervix, or a general anesthetic may be used. The surgeon will extract the fetus and suction curettage will be used to remove the placenta. The procedure may be a D&E (dilatation and extraction) or D&X (a variant of D&E). The D&X procedure is commonly referred to as the *partial-birth abortion,* and is a controversial procedure, both legally and ethically. In l997, the Supreme Court addressed this issue.

Saline injection is performed between the 16th and 24th weeks of gestation. The procedure involves withdrawing between 50 and 200 mL of amniotic fluid through a needle and syringe. Approximately 200 mL of saline solution is then injected slowly into the remaining amniotic fluid. This procedure brings about normal labor and delivery of the fetus within 18 to 20 hours. The same procedure is used to instill prostaglandin into the amniotic sac, except only a small amount of amniotic fluid is removed. The results are the same. These procedures can be performed only in a hospital and require a stay of 1 to 3 days, and are used infrequently due to health risks to the woman.

In a very few cases, a hysterotomy is performed to remove the fetus surgically or a hysterectomy is performed. These procedures are considered major surgeries, requiring hospitalization and a longer period of recuperation than other methods. They usually are performed only in the case of uterine abnormalities.

Generally, the later an abortion of any type is performed, the greater the risk. Psychological and physiological difficulties may accompany any method of abortion. When pregnancy is to be terminated, for any reason, only qualified physicians and appropriate facilities should be used. Women are advised to seek professional help as soon as possible for their own safety and well-being.

IN THE NEWS

On a Planned Parenthood website, a question was asked if having an abortion would negatively affect a woman's ability to have children. The response was that abortions are safe. In fact, abortions are 11 times safer than giving birth if the abortion is performed in the first 12 weeks of pregnancy (90% of abortions are), and there are no unusual complications. It will not affect a woman's ability to have children. The risk for a second abortion is generally the same as for the first abortion if performed within 12 weeks of pregnancy. There is no evidence that having more than one abortion causes any health problems. However, the health risks increase the longer the pregnancy goes on before an abortion is performed.

Legal Implications

In the United States, as states turned away from English common law during the late-18th and early 19th centuries, statutory criminal law began to address abortion. In 1821, Connecticut, and then in 1828, New York, passed abortion laws making post-quickening abortion a felony and pre-quickening abortion a misdemeanor. This process continued through to the 1830s and 1850s respectively. In the 19th century, abortion regulations tightened. By the late-1860s, throughout most of United States, abortions were prohibited except to preserve the life of the mother. Those laws and subsequent ones remained in place until the 1960s and 1970s when many states liberalized their abortion laws.

One of the monumental decisions affecting a change of all abortion laws was the 1973 U.S. Supreme Court *Roe v Wade* decision. Jane Roe (a pseudonym) was a single, pregnant woman who took action against Henry Wade, the District Attorney of Dallas County, in 1970. Roe pleaded the Fourteenth Amendment and her "right to privacy," claiming the Texas antiabortion statute unconstitutional.

As a result, 3 years later the Supreme Court held that during the first trimester, pregnant women have a constitutional right to abortions, and the state has no vested interest in regulating them at that time. During the second trimester, the state may regulate abortion and insist on reasonable standards of medical practice if an abortion is to be performed. During the third trimester, the state interests override pregnant women's rights to abortions, and the state may "proscribe abortion except when necessary to preserve the health or life of the mother."[2]

Although this court decision did "favor" Roe, many unanswered questions resulted. For example, when is the fetus viable? Is the fetus the "property" of the bearer? Does the woman alone have the right, or do husbands, partners, or parents have rights? Can state and federal funding be required for abortions? Virtually every state statute on abortion was invalidated, either partly or totally, by *Roe v Wade*. The public responded to their legislators, who, in turn, reacted through legislation. Some statutes set abortion facility requirements; others required detailed reports on performed abortions and what consultations were required.

In the 1973 *Doe v Bolton* case, the Supreme Court struck down four preabortion procedural requirements: (1) residency, (2) performance of the abortion in a hospital accredited by the Joint Commission on Accreditation of Hospitals (JCAH), (3) approval by a committee of the hospital's medical staff, and (4) consultations. It also had a "conscience clause" stating that physicians and medical employees could refuse to participate in abortions without being discriminated against.

Another U.S. Supreme Court decision in 1976 changed state abortion statutes. The court ruled, on constitutional grounds, that spousal and parental consent is not necessary for an abortion. Currently courts tend not to differentiate between minor and adult pregnant women. Absolute parental consent may force pregnant minors to seek criminal or self-induced abortions. A 1978 U.S. Supreme Court decision held that a state may not constitutionally legislate a blanket, unreviewable power of parents to veto their daughter's abortion.

In June 1977, three related cases, *Beal v Doe, Maher v Roe,* and *Poelker v Doe,* resulted in Supreme Court decisions affecting abortion laws. The ruling stated "the states have neither a constitutional nor a statutory obligation under Medicaid to provide non-therapeutic abortions for indigent women or access to public facilities for the performance of such abortions."

In 1983, the Supreme Court reaffirmed the *Roe v Wade* decision when it heard *Akron v Akron Center for Reproductive Health, Inc.* In Akron, Ohio, three physicians and the center brought suit against the city challenging the constitutionality of city provisions that regulated abortion performance. The city had passed an ordinance requiring that (1) second-trimester abortions be performed in hospitals, (2) specific information be given by physicians to patients undergoing abortion, (3) there be a 24-hour waiting period between consent and performance of the abortion, and (4) there be specific procedures about how physicians were to dispose of the fetal remains. The case was appealed to the U.S. Supreme Court, which found all provisions unconstitutional except for the hospitalization requirement for second-trimester abortions.

Justice Sandra Day O'Connor contended in her dissent in the *Akron* case that "the *Roe* framework, then, is clearly on a collision course with itself. As the medical risks of various abortion procedures decrease, the point at which the State may regulate for reasons of maternal health is moved forward to actual childbirth. As medical science becomes better able to provide for the separate existence of the fetus, the point of viability is moved further back toward conception."

In a similar case in 1986, the U.S. Supreme Court again reaffirmed *Roe v Wade.* In *Thornburgh v American College of Obstetricians and Gynecologists,* the Supreme Court ruled against the following issues: informed consent and printed information that would have required a physician to provide information 24 hours before the abortion related to available medical assistance benefits; the father's liability for assistance; a description of alternatives to abortion; possible detrimental effects not foreseeable; and medical risks of the abortion, as well as of carrying the child to full term.

In addition, the Supreme Court struck down a ruling that would have required physicians to determine whether the fetus was viable and to report to the State Department of Health specific information normally considered private. This information would have included such items as the woman's age, race, and number of pregnancies, marital status, and date of last menses. This information was to be open for public inspection without the woman's name. Third, the Supreme Court ruled against physician involvement in postviability care for the child and the requirement for a second physician at postviability abortions.

In 1991, the U.S. Supreme Court upheld a ban on abortion counseling at federally funded clinics. This ban affects approximately 4000 clinics serving 4.5 million women, mostly with low incomes. The result is that these clinics cannot mention abortion as an option. Some clinics receiving federal funds have chosen to do without the funding so that abortion still can be presented as an option. Many observers think that this ban and the greater issue of abortion will be fought in the political world rather than in the courts.

In July 1992, the U.S. Supreme Court, in *Planned Parenthood v Casey,* ruled that Pennsylvania's requirement that spouses be notified before abortion was an "undue burden."

In *Schenck v Pro-Choice Network,* 519 US 357 (1997), the U.S. Supreme Court addressed the question of whether an injunction that places restrictions on demonstrations outside abortion clinics violates the First Amendment. Health care providers and others wanted to restrict blockades and other disruptive activities in front of abortion clinics. The U.S. District Court created a "fixed-buffer zone" prohibiting demonstrations within 15 feet of entrances into abortion clinics, parking lots, or driveways. The court also created a "floating-buffer zone" prohibiting demonstrators from coming within 15 feet of people or vehicles wishing access to abortion clinics. The U.S. Supreme Court held that the fixed buffer zones were constitutional because they protected the government's right to protect public safety. Floating buffer zones were found unconstitutional because they imposed a greater burden on free speech (First Amendment).

In June 2000, the U.S. Supreme Court ruled on two cases: (1) *Stenberg, Attorney General of Nebraska, et al. v Carhart,* and (2) *Hill et al. v Colorado et al.* Nebraska law prohibits any "partial birth abortion" unless that procedure is necessary to save the mother's life. The definition of partial birth abortion was a procedure in which the doctor partially delivers vaginally a living unborn child before killing the child. Nebraska held that this was a violation of the law, was a felony, and revoked the physician's license. The district court held the statute constitutional. The circuit court affirmed. The U.S. Supreme Court said Nebraska's statute criminalizes the performance of "partial birth abortions" and violates the federal constitution.

In a Colorado case the same year, their state law held it unlawful for any person within 100 feet of a health care facility's entrance to "knowingly approach" within 8 feet of another person in order to pass leaflets/information to that person without that person's consent. The court held that the statute imposed content-neutral time, place, and manner restrictions narrowly tailored to serve a government interest. The state Supreme Court affirmed concluding that the statute was narrowly drawn, concluding that ample alternative channels of communication remained open to petitioners. The U.S. Supreme Court affirmed that the restrictions on speech-related incidences are constitutional.

In 2003, *Scheidler v NOW; Operation Rescue v NOW,* the U. S. Supreme Court dissolved the 10-year permanent injunction prohibiting protesters from demonstrating outside abortion clinics.

In 2006, *Ayotte v Planned Parenthood of Northern New England* challenged the New Hampshire law that requires a parent be notified 48 hours before an abortion is provided to a minor. The Supreme Court held the law unconstitutional because it does not permit an immediate abortion without notifying a parent in medical emergencies that threaten a minor's health.

A number of state lawmakers, disenchanted with *Roe v Wade* and the resultant unsuccessful challenges in the U.S. Supreme Court have begun to take action on their own. South Dakota banned most abortions in that state in direct conflict with the U.S. Supreme Court and with the full intention of creating a constitutional challenge. Even though the governor signed the bill in South Dakota, abortions have not stopped and will not stop until the law passes through all the court challenges stacked up against the constitutionality of the act. There are at least 11 states that are considering banning abortion and more are expected to follow. They include Alabama, Georgia, Indiana, Kentucky, Louisiana, Missouri, Mississippi, Ohio, Oklahoma, Tennessee, and Virginia. Already, agencies such as Planned Parenthood are planning to fight the legislation in the courts.

Other legal challenges continue, and more Supreme Court decisions are expected. The majority of abortion questions arise over the Fourteenth Amendment and the equal protection clause. Every citizen of the United States has "equal protection of the law" and shall not be discriminated against. This includes abortion. The parties are testing the courts on these constitutional issues. For example, is it discriminatory for a woman who has money and insurance coverage to receive an abortion but a woman who is poor and relies on welfare to be

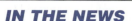

IN THE NEWS

The Senate in July 2006 voted to make it a crime to take a pregnant girl across state lines to obtain an abortion without her parent's knowledge. Many see this as the most significant congressional action in years. Proponents of the bill say it will protect the health and safety of minors and protect the rights of parents. What would opponents say? Forty-four states require either parental consent or notification for a minor to have an abortion. Five states have laws that require both parents' involvement. Oklahoma and Utah require both parental notification and consent.

denied an abortion? Will this withstand the scrutiny of the court on the issue of discrimination? Is there a rational basis for discrimination in the case of an unmarried woman versus a married woman seeking an abortion? Can a state require a married woman to obtain her husband's consent? Can a state require a physician to inform the parents of a juvenile who is undergoing an abortion?

A recent report summed up the uniquely complex intersection of individual rights, public interest, and advances in medical technology:

> *Social response to women's reproductive abilities typically has made their bodies part of the public domain in a way that men's are not. Modern medicine, right in step with this tradition, has made women's wombs even more thoroughly public—its technology renders them open to view, and its science tells us with growing precision how the actions of pregnant women affect the health of fetuses.*[3]

The abortion issue and the abortion law are in a state of flux. Radical changes have occurred during the past 100 years. Who can predict what the next 100 years will bring? The political climate, moral attitudes, advances in medical technology, and impact of current abortion laws will influence the future of abortion.

▲ CRITICAL THINKING EXERCISE

President George W. Bush named two new Supreme Court Justices, John Roberts and Samuel Alito. Any change in the court has the potential for overturning *Roe v Wade*. Discuss the role of the U.S. Supreme Court and the political impact of justices who are appointed by the President for a life term.

Ethical Implications

Three major ethical issues surface in a discussion on abortion. Considering these issues separately is being neither honest nor realistic. The issues are as follows:

1. Are there any reasons to justify abortion?
2. Are current laws regarding abortion consistent, fair, and just?
3. Are abortions an appropriate method of birth control?

Are There Any Reasons to Justify Abortions?

To answer "yes" with no restrictions implies that abortions should be performed on demand and at any time during the pregnancy as long as the procedure is still safe. The viability of the fetus or the circumstances is not an issue to consider. The issue is a woman's right to make a decision on whether, if, or when an abortion is to be performed. The pregnant woman's right is higher than any other. The issue is one of freedom and human rights. Proponents of this theory may be called pro-choice.

To answer "no" without any other consideration is to believe that abortion for any reason is murder. The consideration here is that the fetus is innocent, weak, and helpless, and its right to life should be protected at all costs. These individuals often believe that to allow abortion is to also condone **infanticide.** The rights of the fetus and newborn are paramount to the rights of any others. Proponents of this theory may be called pro-life.

Many individuals stand somewhere in the middle. These are the advocates who believe that abortion is permissible to save the life of the mother **(therapeutic abortion).** This situation receives support from pro-choice individuals. The second situation making abortion permissible and receiving support is in the case of rape or incest. For some, the circumstances determine whether an abortion is performed or the fetus is allowed to survive. This premise considers the rights of both mother and fetus and the rights of any others who may be involved. Most likely, pro-choice individuals also consider the question of when life begins.

One may expect that religion offers a solution to the question of when life begins. In discussing ethical questions, actions of churches are often considered. But there is no consensus or agreement here that settles the issue. A few religious groups propose that abortions be performed only when necessary to save the mother's life. Some religious groups determine a time or establish viability of the fetus for performing abortions. All make an attempt to understand the pain and trauma associated with any decision on abortion.

 When identifying abortion issues, consider the following factors:

1. Economics
2. Age
3. Health
4. Religion
5. Culture

Are Current Laws Regarding Abortions Consistent, Fair, and Just?

This second ethical question may be somewhat easier to answer than the first; however, there is no general agreement on a response here either.

As discussed earlier, laws were consistent in the early 1900s—abortions were illegal. The issue came into full public view in 1973 with the *Roe v Wade* Supreme Court decision. Statutes then changed, and abortion became legal.

 These statutes are inconsistent, however. The Supreme Court's intentionally vague ruling has left the states to interpret and regulate abortions. Much variation

---

IN THE NEWS

An abortion case involving a mentally disabled rape victim polarized Argentina, setting the government against courts in a Roman Catholic nation where terminating pregnancy is mostly illegal. The parents wanted an abortion for their daughter, but law banned abortions except when a woman's life was in danger or a "demented" woman was raped. Lower tribunals denied the parent's request and one judge cited her own religious convictions whereas the Governor of Buenos Aires said, "We are not in a theocracy [a government or community governed by a god or priest]. It is within this disabled rape victim's rights to abort." The woman had the abortion.

remains. There is little agreement on the viability of the fetus or what regulations, if any, are established for physicians and facilities. Therefore, abortion rights in one state may not be the same in another.

The consideration of how abortions are to be funded is even more complex. The 1977 Supreme Court ruling that said states were not required to fund abortions for the indigent woman raises the question of fairness and justice in following the law. Essentially, this ruling has the force of denying an abortion to a woman who is unable to pay for one. The right to choose becomes hinged on the ability to pay. This, in effect, denies personal freedom in a free society that has guaranteed equality under the Fourteenth Amendment. The other side of the coin means that opponents of abortion will pay through their taxes in Medicaid funding for those who choose abortion. Persons who object on this basis also must weigh the costs of a funded abortion against the pregnancy, delivery, and welfare costs of the mother and child.

According to the National Abortion Federation Internet web page, the cost of an early, outpatient abortion is about $300 to $500, whereas a later abortion might be $650 to $1,000. Of course the type of abortion method determines the cost. Hospitalizations cost more. Paying for an abortion usually is not a problem for middle- or upper-income women, however, Medicaid restricts funding for poor women generally and other federally funded medical programs. The hidden costs for all women who seek abortions may be "paid" by themselves, their families, or other taxpayers, whether the woman obtains the abortion or decides to go to term with the pregnancy. It is interesting to note that American Adoptions reports that it costs $12,000 to $24,000 per year to raise a child. Another financial consideration to be faced is the care, support, and institutionalization of infants with severe disabilities born if abortions are not allowed. One cannot hold that abortions are morally wrong and therefore should not be funded without being an advocate of health facilities that provide care for babies who require institutionalization.

Are Abortions an Appropriate Method of Birth Control?

The two highest incidences of "abortions on demand" come from individuals who do not practice birth control because it is not available to them or because it is not convenient. The two groups range in age from 20 to 24 and from 15 to 19, respectively, are white, and are unmarried.

For one reason or another contraception is not practiced, and these pregnant women seek an abortion. This is further complicated by data indicating that some of the same women return for a second or third time for abortions.

Is something amiss in the moral standards of our society that may cause or force a teenager to seek an abortion because she felt too guilty or ashamed to practice contraception? It has taken the fear of AIDS to bring our country to the point where sexuality (and more specifically, contraception) is a topic of national discussion and concern. Yet, for many, perhaps most, this topic is still one of considerable discomfort.

Perhaps the problem has developed because easily accessible abortions have encouraged sexual activity without responsibility. Is information about abortions more readily available than information on contraception? Is sex education, whether in the home or school, adequate? Are parents intentional and realistic about teaching morals? Bringing a new human being into the world is a privilege and a responsibility, and it should not be left to accident as a result of exploitation, fear, or ignorance.

Of interest is the fact that the number of American women obtaining legal abortions has declined. In 2002, the abortion rate decreased to its lowest rate since 1976, according to the U.S. Centers for Disease Control.

Protocol for Health Professionals

Physicians and employees must be knowledgeable and understand their own feelings on abortion. Their personal understanding of abortion will enable them to make a decision before their actual involvement. Legally, employees and physicians cannot be forced to participate in abortions against their wishes. The right to refuse, however, does not authorize the right to judge.

 Physicians and employees who participate in abortions are wise to adhere to the following:

1. Participate only within the law.
2. Provide medical knowledge to clients on the stages of pregnancy, viability of the fetus, and methods of abortion.
3. Obtain written, informed consent.
4. Provide counseling as indicated by the situation.
5. Refer as necessary.
6. Keep records confidential.
7. Seek legal counsel when indicated.
8. Be understanding and compassionate.

Summary

Abortion laws are continually in flux and are constantly challenged. Ethical opinions change and debate moves on. Abortion is one of the longest debated issues and has become increasingly politicized. It involves rights of women and rights of the unborn, which adds to its complexity. It is probably impossible that a resolution will ever satisfy everyone. Health professionals will find it difficult to hold a neutral stand. The law grants rights that are to be protected; yet health professionals also must embrace their personal ethics.

QUESTIONS FOR REVIEW

1. Name the various methods of abortion from 3 to 7 days through the third trimester.

_____

_____

2. List the five theories of when life begins.

_____

_____

3. Discuss the important court cases concerning abortion.

_____

_____

4. List ethical issues of abortion.

_____

_____

CLASSROOM EXERCISES

1. In your own words, describe the process that occurs in fetal development.

2. Prepare a 5-minute speech for laypersons on the methods of abortion.

3. As an individual opposed to all abortions, how would you respond to the following problems?
   a. Pregnancies and resultant births from rape or incest
   b. Unwanted children
   c. Infants with severe birth defects

4. As an individual supporting abortion rights, how would you respond to the following problems?
   a. Abortion as contraception
   b. A late-term abortion for convenience
   c. The right to life versus the right to freedom

5. Where might you refer a client for abortion counseling in your community?

6. In South Dakota, the state's American Indian tribes are considering establishing an abortion clinic on the Pine Ridge Indian Reservation that encompasses 2.7 million acres in southwestern South Dakota. Cecilia Fire Thunder, former nurse and first female president of the Oglala Sioux Tribe said, "As Indian women, we fight many battles. This is just another battle we have to fight." Discuss.

7. Under what conditions can an abortion be performed in your state?

8. Your physician begins to perform abortions and you are not sure you want to participate. After exploring your personal beliefs, what will you do as a professional?

REFERENCES

1. Thompson, JB, and Thompson, HO: Ethics in Nursing. Macmillan, New York, 1981, p 75. This text was used in the original writing of the 4th edition; however, the authors significantly changed the text. We wish to acknowledge the reference. Lauersen, N, and Whitney, S: It's Your Body: A Woman's Guide to Gynecology. Berkley Books, New York, 1983, pp 282–300.
2. Furrow, BR, et al: Health Law, Vol 2. West St. Paul, Minn., 2000, pp 376–391.
3. Nelson, JL: The maternal-fetal dyad: Exploring the two-patient obstetric model. Hastings Cent Rep 22(1): 13, 1992.

WEB RESOURCES

▲ America's Adoption Agency www.americanadoptions.com
▲ Answers.com (dilation and extraction) www.answers.com
▲ Center for Disease Control www.cdc.gov
▲ National Right to Life www.nrlc.org/abortion
▲ Planned Parenthood Federation of America Inc. www.plannedparenthood.org

CHAPTER 15

Life and Death

66 *Life is not measured by the number of breaths we take, but by the moments that take our breath away.* 99

Author unknown

LEARNING OBJECTIVES

Upon successful completion of this chapter, you will be able to:

1. Define key terms.
2. Describe the living will, the advance directive, and durable power of attorney for health care.
3. Appraise components of the Patient Self-Determination Act.
4. Restate choices an individual might have in death.

5. Review at least three advances in technology that enhance or prolong life.
6. Describe *euthanasia* and discuss its common usage.
7. Differentiate among various legal definitions of death.
8. Describe two famous court cases and their impact on prolonging life.
9. Express possible legal implications of life-and-death decisions.
10. Discuss at least three ethical implications of life-and-death decisions.
11. Define the role of the health professional in dealing with clients and families in life-and-death decisions.

Vignette: *What happened to my plan?*

Ted is 76 years old. He is retired and lives with his wife of 44 years and their adult daughter. As a laborer, he spent most of his working years with heavy equipment and cranes on land, tugs, and ships. He loves the water. From his home, he sees the Puget Sound and watches the passing ships. Ted has been diagnosed with emphysema and suspected asbestosis. More than 7 years after diagnosis, his breathing is now difficult. His sense of humor, his love of family, his care for others, and his knowledge of the passing ships is as keen as ever.

Ted and his internist are friends. They worship in the same church. When Ted sees his doctor, they tell jokes and swap stories before getting down to the serious business of his illness. Ted refuses using oxygen until he can no longer sleep peacefully. Even then, he uses oxygen only at night. Ted and his wife, Ann, discuss a living will; they talk with their children, and meet with their attorney to update wills and have the Washington State physicians' directive executed. Ted shares it with his physician, and they agree on his care management.

It is a cold and gloomy December. There is rain and even some snow in the Pacific Northwest. Ted is house bound most of the time now. He has little desire to get out. The weather makes his breathing more labored. He is having severe headaches. When Ann suggests Ted visit his doctor, Ted grumbles that there is nothing more the doctor can do. One evening, Ted is unable to wear even his slippers because his feet and legs are so swollen. The water retention makes his feet feel like water pads. In his humor he comments, "I feel like Jesus—walking on water."

Early the next morning, Ted cannot breathe. He is suffocating. Ann dials 911. In minutes emergency medical technicians are at the door. In their quick assessment, they comment on how strong Ted's heart is but how weak his lungs are. Ann explains the emphysema and suspected asbestosis. Ted is transported to the hospital, treated in the emergency room, and moved to intensive care. Ann, their daughter, and their son are at his bedside. Although his breathing is now stabilized, the medical staff inquires about the use of a respirator and a living will. The family responds positively. The physician's directive is later supplied to the hospital.

Circumstances in the next few days greatly alter Ted's life. Ted's physician suffers his own tragedy and is called to Denmark for a family death. When attempts to remove Ted's excess fluid are not totally successful, a nephrologist is called who orders the placement of a shunt in Ted's shoulder for dialysis. Neither Ted nor the family is anxious to begin dialysis. Ted had watched a close and dear friend suffer greatly, lose a limb, and eventually die after years of dialysis. Ted believes that dialysis will make it next to impossible for him to have a "good death." The nephrologist insists and discusses options with the family. "This is just a 'jump start' to get your kidneys going; we will only have to dialyze you twice probably." Ted and

Ann discuss dialysis. There is hesitation, but the decision is finally made. When the consent for dialysis is signed, both Ted and Ann are concerned about all the side effects. The chaplain explains why the form has to list all the possible side effects, even though few if any are likely to occur. Dialysis will begin the next morning.

The family goes home for a night's rest before their return to the hospital early the next morning. The weather, however, intervenes; heavy snow falls during the night. The hills of Seattle are clogged with vehicles going nowhere. Freeways are treacherous. Even the streets to the hospital are impassable. Dialysis technicians and portable dialysis machines are delayed. Their load backs up and patients more critical than Ted wait long past their dialysis time for treatment. Ted's condition worsens. Fortunately, the weather moderates, and dialysis begins. It does little to help, however. After two treatments, Ted begins to bleed internally, and his laboratory tests indicate that an emergency exists. A surgeon is called in—another stranger to the family, but the "freshest" one available. It seems every surgeon and every hospital is overburdened this Christmas holiday. Emergency surgery is scheduled for 5 p.m. The family is at the bedside, but the operating room is full; a **Code Red** in the room Ted is to use delays surgery further. Ted's condition is so critical that the surgeon checks nearby hospitals for an operating room. None is available. Finally at 1 a.m., Ted goes into surgery. The family is told that there is only a 50–50 chance he will survive.

Ted's survives 4 hours of surgery but is returned to the intensive care unit (ICU) on a respirator. There was a bowel perforation and half his colon was removed. He is critical, but amazingly is able to be weaned from his respirator in 24 hours. By now Ted is receiving food and hydration, blood, platelets, antibiotics, and pain medication intravenously. He cannot speak, but is somewhat alert. He is seriously weakened. Urine output decreases and the question of dialysis returns. At this point, all persons involved in Ted's care meet to discuss treatment; they meet with the family. Each family member is interviewed separately about their wishes and Ted's wishes regarding extraordinary means. Earlier an ICU nurse told the family that if even one of them has any hesitation about treatment, the hospital will not follow Ted's wishes. After completion of the interviews, it is clear that the family intends to follow Ted's wishes. Dialysis will cease. It is only a matter of time now. The nephrologist, however, has other ideas. When she discovers dialysis has been discontinued, she demands to know why. When the family explains, she says, "I was not present for that consultation. I will have to hear it from Ted himself." She goes to Ted's bedside, asks him if he can understand her, and says, "Ted, do you want dialysis?" Ted, in his hospital bed with head and shoulders elevated 10 to 20 degrees, has his arms immobilized at his side for the drip of numerous IV lines. An oxygen mask covers his nose and mouth. His eyes show lack of rest and sleep, fear about what is happening to him, and concern for his family. Ted shrugs his shoulders and opens his hands palms upward in gesture. The nephrologist is ordering a chest x-ray and dialysis when the family intervenes. An on-call physician and the nephrologist argue outside Ted's room, in earshot of the family. The attending physician indicates that in Ted's condition, dialysis probably will do more harm than good. His body cannot withstand dialysis. The nephrologist disagrees.

When there seems no hope and the family is feeling powerless, their family physician returns from Denmark and intervenes on behalf of the family. The damage has already been done, however. Ted has suffered not just one but all of the possible side affects the family feared. Ted is now bleeding internally from almost every organ of his body. All IVs are removed except what is needed to keep Ted comfortable. Every breath is the hardest work his body has ever known. Each member of his family says good-bye and tells Ted how much he is loved. Nurses and doctors, so attentive in the previous 25 days, also stop by. The ICU nurses continue to do what they are best known for—attending to the needs of the critically ill. The primary care physician remains close. The end is peaceful. The end is relief—relief from agony and pain, relief from any more difficult decisions, relief from the disappointment that a loved one's wishes were so hard to carry out.

Choices in Life

Throughout the text, many discussions of rights have surfaced both in the legal and the bioethical sections. The right to health care, right to abortion, right to fertility choices, and right to privacy are just a few rights we claim for ourselves. The dialogue continues. Is health care a right or privilege? Is the right or privilege to a few or to everyone? Is the right to abortion ethical? Should fertility choices be available to anyone? How do we protect the right to confidentiality?

We continually make choices in life. What is our quality of the life? Who decides what health care we receive? Does ageism influence health care? Is vulnerability an issue? A child born with physical disabilities can be tormented by peers who tease and taunt. People living in the ghetto projects struggle daily with life issues. An elderly person living alone with no car and no relatives close fears the loss of physical control and independence. Some elderly persons lose their mental and emotional capabilities as well. Some individuals respond to life's challenges with grace, strength, and a happy disposition no matter what life gives them. Others may only be able to face life's challenges with awkwardness, weakness, and an unhappy outlook. As health care professionals, we must remember our clients' vulnerabilities and their circumstances. We need to understand and accept them where they are and provide personalized health care.

Living Wills, Advance Directives, and the Patient Self-Determination Act

Competent adults have always had the right to make choices about their health care, especially the right to forego life-sustaining treatments when death is imminent. Life-prolonging technology, however, advanced further and faster than did health professionals' ability to deal with those advances. Incompetent adults also needed to be able to voice their choices in dying.

More and more often, health care professionals, especially physicians, found themselves in legal and ethical dilemmas with little or no direction from the legal community. Across the country, states began to pass legislation that gave clients the legal right to forego life-sustaining treatments, nutrition, and hydration and provided protection to physicians and hospitals carrying out such orders. Such directives allow individuals or their representatives to make decisions regarding their dying.

California and Washington were forerunners in such legislation. California's document was the **living will;** Washington's response to the legal dilemma was the **physicians' directive,** or Natural Death Act (Fig. 15–1). In addition, the federal government passed the **Patient Self-Determination Act,** which became effective December 1, 1991.

This law applies to all health care institutions receiving payments from Medicare and Medicaid. These institutions include hospitals, skilled nursing facilities, hospices, home care programs, and health maintenance organizations. Physicians become involved when their practice interacts with these institutions.

The Patient Self-Determination Act requires that all adult persons who receive medical care from such institutions be given written information about their right to accept or refuse medical or surgical treatment. These clients must also be given information about their right to formulate advance directives such as living wills and to designate someone to act on their behalf in making health care decisions (**durable power of attorney for health care,** or medical proxy) (see Appendix II).

The actual implementation of the Patient Self-Determination Act remained a matter for the states. In 1992, Pennsylvania became the 50th state to enact advance directive legislation. The Patient Self-Determination Act, however, does not override any state law allowing a health care provider to object on the basis of conscience in the implementation of such an advance directive.

There is a need for better availability and tracking of advance directives as well as a more uniform document for use across the United States. States are establishing secured, web-based registries where legal documents identifying end-of-life wishes for individuals can be stored. Health professionals will be able to retrieve information from the registry to help them make decisions related to their clients. A discussion with physicians of a client's directive should occur prior to its potential use. Clients who take the time to create an advance directive want their wishes implemented.

Durable Power of Attorney for Health Care

In addition to living wills or physicians' directives, many individuals choose to use the durable power of attorney or the durable power of attorney for health care, legal documents that add another dimension to the decision-making process. Although the living will or physicians' directive allows the writer

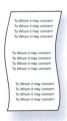

Living Will

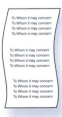

Physicians' Directives

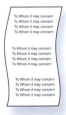

Durable Power of Attorney for Health Care

FIGURE 15–1 Three types of legal documents that communicate patients' choices about their health care.

to determine whether heroic or extraordinary measures will be used, the durable power of attorney allows an agent to act on an individual's behalf in additional ways.

The durable power of attorney is a legal form that allows a designated person to act on another's behalf. Likewise, the durable power of attorney for health care or the medical proxy more specifically allows a designated person to make only health care decisions for another. This proxy or person becomes an agent, or attorney-in-fact. This agent may be a spouse, partner, grown child, close friend, or other relative or someone in whom the person has full confidence. A person must be competent to sign a power of attorney. Some states require that the signer must be able to manage his or her own property effectively at the time of signing. The reason for signing a power of attorney is to ensure that someone will be around to act for a person who becomes physically or mentally disabled. The signer keeps control over the signed legal form as long as the person can manage independently. The signed document can be given to a lawyer or a close friend with instructions that it should not be turned over to the attorney-in-fact unless the need arises. Once signed, the document is in effect until it is revoked.

The designated person who acts on behalf of the client should know and understand the client's living will. What would happen if the power of attorney acted in violation of the client's living will? No court has taken action to see who would prevail. Thus it is wise to ensure that the power of attorney will act on the client's behalf in all instances of health care.

Each state has established rules governing the use of the durable power of attorney. It is best to periodically update and review a durable power of attorney as well as the advance directive. Also, it is best to review each state's laws if moving from state to state. This is an example of when a nationwide registry would ensure client's wishes are followed. Professional legal advice regarding a given state's stipulations and requirements may be advisable, but preprinted forms are readily available. See Appendix II for an example of a durable power of attorney for health care.

Choices in Dying

In dying, what choices are there? How many of the choices in dying are personal decisions; how many are regulated or controlled by technology and advanced medicine? The vignette of Ted helps identify some of the difficulties in decision-making.

Personal attitudes and public opinion have changed through the years. For example, in 1938 the Euthanasia Society of America was founded. It was a national, nonprofit organization dedicated to fostering communication about complex end-of-life decisions among individuals. The organization is best known for inventing the living will in 1967. Today there are numerous organizations dedicated to choices in dying such as Compassion in Choices, The National Hospice and Palliative Care Organization, World Federation of Right to Die Societies, and Death with Dignity National Center.

Individuals are increasingly seeking control over choices in dying; however, the power, the almost coercive power of medical technology and medicine to preserve and prolong life may cause many to suffer years of debility, pain, and perhaps a lesser quality of life.

The desire to have choices in dying comes from fears and concerns related to prolonged dying as the result of technological interventions. Most desire to be able to refuse treatment or hospitalization. Some might choose assisted suicide. Generally, individuals do not want to be a burden to significant others. They may fear becoming senile and dependent. Some may fear loss of control and want to choose their quality of life and have the choice of how they die. Medical technology offers insulin to control diabetes, a cardiac pacemaker or mechanical heart valves for a weak or diseased heart, renal dialysis for kidney failure, and angioplasty for clogged arteries.

Every day, medical personnel are confronted with more complex issues regarding the meanings of life and death. Where is the fine line between helping a person to live and allowing him or her to die? When is it appropriate to use extraordinary means to prolong life? What are extraordinary means? What are the legal implications if physicians withhold or withdraw treatment? Is there a difference between human need and human right? Who decides?

Each of us will die. From the moment we are born, we begin to die. Each day of life moves us closer to our death. Some of us will die suddenly and peacefully, perhaps in our sleep. Some of us will die suddenly as a result of an accident or as a victim of crime. Some of us will die slowly and gradually, with our bodies deteriorating and our organs ceasing to function. Some of us will die with little or no pain or discomfort. Some of us will die after great pain and discomfort. Most of us want to live, but when faced with death, we desire to go quickly, painlessly, and with dignity. However, not all of us will be so fortunate.

Many who would be dead are alive because of technological or mechanical intervention. Of the more than 2.4 million annual deaths in the United States, more than half will occur in health care facilities. And of those deaths, most are preceded by some deliberate decision to stop or not start medical treatment.

Consider the following example from Donald M. Hayes[1] writing in *Between Doctor and Patient:*

> *Mr. Baker had terminal kidney failure and was comatose. Several tubes came from various places in his body. He was receiving both blood and glucose into his veins. One night he went into cardiac arrest. A team of nurses and physicians responded to a "Code Red" and worked vigorously to resuscitate. The attempt was futile and Mr. Baker died. The memory of Mr. Baker's death was lasting to Mr. Rogers, the recently admitted patient in the same room. He said to his physician, "Please don't ever let that happen to me. I've tried all my life to live like a man; I want to die like one." Mr. Rogers underwent surgery that revealed inoperable, widespread cancer. He did not respond well, and a few days later he had a tube in his stomach, a catheter in his bladder, a tube through his nose, and intravenous tubes in both arms. When he suffered respiratory failure, a tracheotomy was performed to save his life. He was given a slate to write on, since a tracheotomy precludes speech. Later one evening, before he managed to switch off this respirator so that he might die peacefully, he wrote on the slate, "Doctor, remember; the enemy is not death. The enemy is inhumanity."*

Few for whom life has meaning would turn their backs on the medical technology that has added years of life for so many. Such advances in medicine are heralded by the public and the media; however, if not used judiciously, technology can supplant the quality of life. Technology has heightened our awareness of death at the same time that it increases our life span.

At some time in our lives, each of us will face the issue of how much medical technology to use to prolong life. Perhaps, too, we will wish for a "good death." Whether or not to prolong life may become a serious problem when the decision may be made with little forethought or adequate planning. When the physician tells a loved one that a cardiac pacemaker is necessary to regulate the heartbeat, the general response is "When can it be done?"

The decision is more complex; however, when the loved one is hospitalized with a heart condition that is rapidly deteriorating and little can be done. The questions of how much intervention and when are much more serious. When the heart monitor indicates with a buzz and a continuous monotone sound that the heart has ceased to beat, somewhere, someone is going to ask, "Do we resuscitate?" It is at this point that the decisions declared in a living will or durable power of attorney for health care become significant especially when family and health care providers are informed.

▲ CRITICAL THINKING EXERCISE

Refer to the preceding example of Mr. Baker and Mr. Rogers. What would you do if you were the physician? What would you do if you were a loved one? Would your actions cause any difficulties? If so, describe.

Each of us wants to control his or her life, especially when it comes to our own dying. Maintaining that control may be more easily envisioned and said than done. There may be many choices to make. We truly want a "good death" as much as we want a "good life." Given the ultimate power over choice, we would choose the good death, or **euthanasia.**

To use the term *euthanasia* in this context, however, is not so common today. Euthanasia has come to refer only to the active form, in which some action causes the death of another. This is in contrast to what might be called passive euthanasia, or the use of deliberate decisions that may result in death.

For example, are antibiotics prescribed when a hospitalized person contracts pneumonia and is suffering from the last stages of pancreatic cancer? Under what circumstances are "do not resuscitate" orders placed in clients' charts at hospitals or long-term-care facilities?

Another person is being kept alive by a respirator. The client has no recognition and no awareness of surroundings. After careful assessment of the situation and a discussion and agreement with the family members, the medical staff turns off the equipment. Life support ceases. In a matter of minutes, the heart monitor indicates a flat line rather than a heartbeat. Death occurs.

How much pain medication will be prescribed for a client? If sufficient pain medication is prescribed to keep those close to death comfortable, health professionals know the medication provided for pain relief may depress breathing in some clients already so debilitated that death is hastened.

To ensure that we have choices in dying, all 50 states have passed legislation that allows us to make choices in death and to dictate to health care professionals our wishes.

▲ CRITICAL THINKING EXERCISE

"When I am dying, I am quite sure that the central issues for me will not be whether I am put on a ventilator, whether CPR is attempted when my heart stops, or whether I receive artificial feeding. Although each of these could be important, each will almost certainly be quite peripheral. Rather, my central concerns will be how to face my death, how to bring my life to a close, and how best to help my family go on without me. A ventilator will not help me do these things—not unless all I need is a little more time to get the job done." Unfortunately, however, bioethics has succumbed to the agendas of physicians. Physicians face ethical concerns about treatment decisions regarding when to offer, withhold, and withdraw various treatments and treatment decisions have been the focus of bioethics as well. But the issues that most trouble patients and their families at the end of life are not these. To them, the end of life is a spiritual crisis.[2] Discuss.

Legal Definitions of Death

An early legal definition of death was the cessation of the heart and lung wherein the two were so interrelated that the cessation of one leads to the cessation of another, followed by the cessation of all cognitive activity, all other brain functions, and all responsiveness in general. The cessation of the heart and of breathing was the simplest to identify and the easiest test of life, and it became the acceptable definition of death. Today, the majority of deaths in the United States are determined by this traditional definition of death.

With medical technological advances, resuscitative devices, increased complexities of life, and organ transplants, the heart–lung definition of death was found insufficient. Death is a continuum, and different parts of the body die at different times. The heart may stop before or after the client dies. For example, in a heart attack victim, the heart stops beating, but the client does not die immediately. Approximately 3 to 4 minutes pass before there is irreparable brain death. At this point, the client is dead. Once the brain dies, there is no need for the other body organs, and they die at various intervals.

Subsequently, the concept of brain death was presented by the Harvard Ad-Hoc Committee, chaired by Henry Beecher. The criteria were simple: A client in this state appears to be in deep coma. The condition can be satisfactorily diagnosed by the following points: (1) unreceptivity and unresponsivity, (2) no movements or breathing, (3) no reflexes, and (4) a flat electroencephalogram. Each of these tests shall be repeated at least 24 hours later with no change.[3] This definition of brain death does not cover cases such as Karen Ann Quinlan, who was in a persistent vegetative state, or people who are in comas but do not meet other accepted criteria.

In 1983, President Ronald Reagan formed a commission to discuss the ethical implications of dying and death. The commission's report, entitled "Deciding to Forego Life-Sustaining Treatment," recommended that all U.S. jurisdictions accept the Uniform Determination of Death Act. The act was developed under the commission's direction by three organizations: the American Bar Association, the American Medical Association, and the National Conference of Commissioners on Uniform State Laws. The act "established that the irreversible cessation of all circulatory and respiratory functions, or irreversible cessation of all functions of the entire brain, including the brain stem" is the criterion of death.[4] The commission further stated that such a definition ought to incorporate general physiological standards rather than medical criteria or tests that would change with advances in medical technology.

Some believe that the higher brain death definition addresses all purposes. This definition is the permanent and irreversible cessation of all higher brain or neocortical functions. In recent years, bioethicists and philosophers have criticized the brain death criteria because even after a standard battery of tests for brain death, many brain functions persist. It is recognized, too, that medical technology and improved diagnostic skill has moved the time of death closer to when death actually occurs. The higher brain death definition may allow a greater allowance of who is "dead," and would allow those with cognitive impairments to be declared dead.

Whatever the state's legal definition of death, the declaration of death will be made by medical standards as defined in the Uniform Determination of Death Act. This means that as technology changes and medicine advances, laws will not necessarily change; rather, good medical practices will determine what counts as good evidence that the legal definition of death has occurred. With the heart–lung definition, there may be some leeway on the part of the physician to determine death. For example, if a relative is traveling to the dying client, the physician may choose to keep the client alive until the relative says good-bye. Further, when a physician declares a person dead, that physician should not be involved in the transplantation of organs, although this is not required by law. Transplantation is discussed in Chapter 16.

Legal Implications

Most legal rulings on life and death center on "Who makes the decisions?" Prolonging life by artificial means usually poses few legal problems. Federal laws state that kidney clients have the right to funding and the use of kidney dialysis machines. Some means of prolonging life artificially, such as insulin administration, are so easy, inexpensive, and widely practiced that there is no controversy about their use. On the other hand, some procedures, such as dialysis, are so expensive that federal legislation was necessary to ensure that every citizen has the right to such treatments regardless of cost.

Choices in dying, however, are complex and controversial. Consider landmark case law in the following two circumstances. In seeking greater choice in the process of dying, the courts appear to be regulating in a more restrictive manner. Is litigation the reason why health care professionals and institutions sometimes do not want to abide by clients' choices in dying? Is there a general feeling that we do indeed have rights, but the right to die or to make our own choices about dying is not so carefully protected?

Karen Ann Quinlan: The litigation over the case of Karen Ann Quinlan was widely publicized. Quinlan was a New Jersey woman who, at age 21, was taken to the hospital in a comatose state by friends after a birthday party. No one is sure exactly what happened to Karen on Tuesday, April 14, 1975, but the world soon began to follow her life closely. Her case was a newsworthy first. Karen's condition deteriorated. On July 31, her parents gave her physicians permission to take Karen off the respirator and signed a letter to that effect. The physicians disagreed with the decision on moral grounds and refused to take Karen off the respirator. Legal action ensued. On September 12, the attorney for Joseph Quinlan, Karen's father, filed a plea with the superior court on three constitutional grounds: (1) the right to privacy, (2) religious freedom, and (3) cruel and unusual punishment.

Judge Robert Muir ruled against Joseph Quinlan, who then appealed the decision to the New Jersey Supreme Court. The court's decision was in Joseph Quinlan's favor and set aside any criminal liability for removing the respirator. It further recommended that Karen's physicians consult the hospital ethics committee to concur with their prognosis for Karen. Weeks later Karen was weaned from the machine. She lived until 1986.

Theresa (Terri) Schiavo: Terri Schiavo suffered cardiac arrest in February 1990, probably due to an eating disorder that may have caused a serious electrolyte imbalance diagnosed when she was admitted to the hospital. She was without oxygen 5 to 7 minutes longer than medical experts believe is possible without irreversible brain damage. Her husband, Michael, insisted she be intubated, given a tracheotomy to breathe, and placed on a respirator. Without these actions, she would have died. Terri lived in a coma for 2 months and then was repeatedly diagnosed as in a persistent vegetative state. She was removed from the respirator and kept functioning with an artificial feeding and hydration tube. She could breathe and swallow her saliva, but could not drink or eat. What happened in the next 15 years is almost unimaginable.

Terri's husband and her parents struggled for a few years, but conflict arose when Michael and her parents disagreed about removing the feeding tube so Terri could die peacefully. Terri had no living will. Twice courts ordered the feeding tube to be removed, but Terri's parents fought to have it reinserted. The Florida legislature passed a law known as "Terri's Law" to give the governor the prerogative of reinserting the feeding tube and required a special guardian ad litem be appointed. Later, the Florida Supreme Court ruled Terri's Law unconstitutional, and the U.S. Supreme Court refused to overturn that decision. Just a week prior to Terri's death, the U.S. Congress passed legislation to move the case from Florida to the federal courts. The Florida Federal District Court, the 11th Circuit Court of Appeals and the U.S. Supreme Court refused to review the findings of the lower courts.

By this time and through all the court battles, Michael and Terri's parents were estranged and could no longer be civil toward each other. In testimony, Terri's parents said that even if Terri had a living will, they would have fought to have it voided. Michael became even more determined to carry out the wishes he believed Terri would have wanted. In the last few days of Terri's life, private citizens, religious leaders, and news media lined up on both sides of the issue outside the hospital to witness a most public death. Michael's wishes finally prevailed and Terri died March 31, 2005, 14 days after the feeding tube was removed and 15 years following her cardiac arrest.

In the more than 30 years since the Quinlan case, similar cases have caused emotional trauma to families faced with the death of a loved one. The case of Schiavo drew as much national attention, if not more, than the Quinlan case. Both cases provoked discussions about end-of-life issues and medicine's limitations. Both Quinlan and Schiavo were alive when their cases were brought before the courts. The question in both cases was whether each woman should be kept alive, one by use of a respirator, the other by receiving artificial hydration and nutrition. It was not whether they were legally dead. Their families were asking questions. "Should they be allowed to die?" "Is vegetative existence better than death?" What do you think? What impact should medical technology have on these decisions? Who pays? Who should decide? Is it more difficult to remove hydration and nutrition than a respirator?

▲ CRITICAL THINKING EXERCISE

A healthy 37-year-old woman was found to be anemic during a yearly physical exam. She was advised to eat foods high in iron. Three months later she again saw her physician because she was so exhausted. Her physician performed lab tests and a colonoscopy and called her back in for an appointment. He said to her, "The tumor we found was malignant. I'm sorry to tell you, you have colon cancer in its advanced stages." She doesn't remember the rest of the office visit. Discuss.

Ethical Considerations

Life-and-death choices are numerous. The many factors to consider include the following: Who makes the decision? What role do politicians and the courts play in making life-and-death decisions. What is the influence of economics? What about the insurance companies? Whose right is paramount—the client's or the health care provider's or someone else? Do circumstances influence decisions? If so, what are they? What is ordinary and extraordinary treatment? Should resuscitation be started? Should treatment be withheld?

Who makes the decision is not easy to determine. Clients like to believe they do. Many times physicians alone decide. Other times, it is determined by the institutions where people are being treated. The government, through state statutes, may determine who shall live or die. The burden of such decisions is heavy. If a decision is required in an emergency life-and-death matter, those in closest proximity to the client will decide.

In health care facilities, the law may determine who decides. A main function of such facilities is to preserve life. If there is any question, consideration is given to the wishes of the client, the wishes of the family, the recommendations of the physician, and perhaps the recommendations of a professional team of individuals whose purpose it is to make a decision—not necessarily in that order.

The problem arises over whose right is paramount in a decision. At times it is obvious. If a client is unable to decide, for whatever reason, others have to be involved. The family has an influence. The cases of Karen Ann Quinlan and Theresa Schiavo demonstrated that the influence of family is not decisive, however. In the case of Theresa Schiavo, the governor of

Florida, the 11th Circuit Court of Appeals, the Florida Supreme Court, the President of the United States, Congress, and the United States Supreme Court were all involved.

The same often is true of a client's wishes. Even if clients are able to express their wishes to physicians and health care providers, circumstances may override them.

Consider, for example, an elderly client with a physician's directive who communicates that he wishes to die at home. He nears death and has difficulty breathing. His family members call emergency help. Paramedics, of necessity and training, use heroic measures to prevent death and then transport the client to the nearest hospital. In this case, it is best for family members to recognize that such actions may circumvent the client's choice and the physician's directive.

Many circumstances influence decisions. Age is a factor. Resuscitation may be started on a 16-year-old and not on an 89-year-old. Cost is also a factor. Triple cardiac bypass surgery may be performed for someone of substantial means more readily than for the indigent derelict. Health is a factor. A pacemaker may be inserted for the elderly client whose general health is good, but it may not be used if the client's health is poor and other severe physical difficulties exist. The availability of resources is a factor. With only one kidney and four needy persons, three will have to do without.

Other factors include region, personal philosophy of life, the amount of pain one can endure, whether a client is comatose, and what the client's feelings are on a good life versus a good death. All of these factors are relative. Some are old at age 45; others are young at 90. Some can endure great pain, and others have a low threshold for pain. What is poor health to one person may seem to be good health to another. The relativity of the factors complicates the decision and mandates that each decision be considered individually on its own merits.

REMEMBER... No one ethical guideline is adequate for a statement on choices in dying.

One ethical view is that euthanasia is murder because of either omission or commission. Tied closely with this view are some religious beliefs that only God has the right to decide at what moment a person should die and that euthanasia violates the command "Thou shall not kill." Some religious groups believe suffering is part of the divine plan for every person; others believe that their faith cannot possibly tolerate a bad death for anyone.

The possibility also exists that clients pronounced incurable may recover, which would be impossible if euthanasia already had been committed. Clients suffering greatly may request to die on the spur of the moment with little thought of the ramifications.

According to the American Medical Association's Council on Ethical and Judicial Affairs, physicians are discouraged from engaging in any form of euthanasia because it is seen as fundamentally incompatible with their role of healer. It is recommended that physicians aggressively facilitate the needs of dying clients by giving pain medication, offering emotional support, respecting clients' autonomy, and having good communication. Interestingly, too, medical schools increasingly are teaching students to deal with the dying client—that heroic saving of life is only half of their job.

Some people believe that legal euthanasia or physician-assisted suicide would weaken the moral fiber of the country and may lead to such actions for eugenic reasons. If we can justify death for one individual to prevent further suffering, why not for infants with severe disabilities who have no possibility of a "normal" life? Consider the circumstances of an infant born with severe congenital defects and intestinal obstructions requiring surgery. The medical staff and parents may decide not to operate and let the infant die. Allowing this to occur is not easy. It means watching a tiny infant gradually dehydrate and suffer from infection, perhaps for a period of days. The ordeal can be terrible. Parents are protected from this experience, but the medical staff is not. Many physicians and health professionals ask, "Would it

---

IN THE NEWS

Cultures view life and death differently. For example, people of Jewish heritage strive to appreciate each day and live it as though it is their last. Death is seen as a part of the life cycle. Mexicans also view death as a natural part of life and the will of God. In the Filipino culture, planning one's death is taboo, hence, discussing advanced directives and living wills is difficult. Many Chinese believe their spirits do not rest unless living descendants care for the grave and worship the memory of the dead. In the Japanese culture, family members want to be by the dying person's bedside and traditionally the eldest son has decision-making responsibility at this time. There is, however, a taboo against the discussion of serious illness and death. Being aware of one's cultural perspective and asking questions related to their wishes is better than assuming everyone thinks and believes alike.

---

not be more merciful to inject the infant with a lethal dose of medication that would cause death to come quickly and painlessly and prevent the suffering?"

Perhaps even more personal and difficult questions are "How do I want to die?" "What kind of lifesaving measures would I want?" "Do I prefer active euthanasia or physician-assisted suicide?" "Can I stand to suffer?" "Do I have any control over my own death?" "Do I have a right to die as I choose?" "What would I want health professionals to do for me?"

The Role of Health Professionals in Health Care

Health care employees will make life-and-death decisions in personal relationships with their families and friends, but rarely in any professional capacity. They often, however, may be involved in conversations with clients or their families who are struggling with the question. They also may be sounding boards to physicians involved in the decision-making process. Certainly the law should be followed, religious and cultural practices considered, and the clients' rights protected when possible, but no clearly established guideline is available.

Clients who willingly and openly discuss their beliefs and wishes concerning their own deaths should be encouraged to complete living wills or physicians' directives and durable power of attorney documents. Legal counsel should be recommended to people if appropriate. Clients should not be made to feel ashamed or guilty because of their feelings about death, no matter how much they differ from your personal feelings.

Health professionals must be understanding and compassionate. Every attempt must be made to respect the feelings of clients and their families. Families should be allowed to express any guilt they may feel in making decisions. A clear picture of the circumstances, explained by the physician in words clients can comprehend, can alleviate much of that problem. Clients who have strong feelings about having their lives prolonged should be encouraged to make their wishes known.

When health professionals are confronted with situations or questions they cannot handle, consultations and referrals should be sought. Attorneys may be called, and medical societies may offer assistance. Hospital ethics committees may be valuable. Hospital chaplains, staff psychiatrists, and social workers are specially trained to help others with these personal and processional issues. Decisions of the kind discussed in this chapter weigh heavily on the minds of those involved. That weight should not be allowed to become too great.

▲ CRITICAL THINKING EXERCISE

Websites listed at the end of the chapter have advance directives specific to each state. Download your state's advanced directive and durable power of attorney. Discuss what you would do with this information both as an individual and as a health professional.

Summary

Choices about dying are best made while living whenever possible. Legal documents should be executed and shared with loved ones, family members, and health professionals in order to ensure that personal wishes are followed. These choices are not easily made unless there is a willingness to discuss the issue of death and what measures are to be taken when dying. If death can be viewed as another stage in life, even if the final one, it will be easier to have this discussion. Health professionals are bound to abide by the wishes of their clients within legal parameters.

QUESTIONS FOR REVIEW

1. List the uses of the
   a. Advance directive.

_____

_____

_____

   b. Patient Self-Determination Act.

_____

_____

_____

   c. Durable power of attorney for health care.

_____

_____

_____

2. Define the
a. Harvard Ad-Hoc Committee definition of death.

_____

_____

_____

b. Uniform Determination of Death Act.

_____

_____

_____

3. List at least three legal implications in life-and-death decisions.

_____

_____

_____

4. Name at least two ethical considerations in life-and-death decisions.

_____

_____

_____

CLASSROOM QUESTIONS

1. If you knew you would be put in the same situation as Karen Ann Quinlan or Terri Schiavo, what would you wish? Why?

2. Identify procedures that prolong life that you would be willing to have. Identify those you would not choose and justify your responses.

3. A family member comes to the ambulatory health care setting. She is angry because the hospital "won't stop their endless testing" and "keeps trying the impossible with my husband." What is your response?

4. A surgical client with a guarded prognosis initiates a conversation with the physician: "If I'm not going to make it, don't let me suffer." How can the physician respond?

5. Under what circumstances might physicians and family members choose not to initiate heroic measures for a client?

6. How would you deal with the situation if you were a nurse in a hospital nursery in which orders from the medical staff and family indicate "do not feed" for an infant with serious birth defects?

7. How would you feel about a husband who follows his wife's request for euthanasia? The husband is not sure he has made the right decision, and his adult children are critical of his decision.

8. In the case of Ted, in which conflict that arose among Ted, the family, and the medical professionals, where did the power ultimately reside? Explain your answer. Discuss your personal reaction to Ted's case. What went right and what went wrong?

REFERENCES

1. Hayes, DM: Between Doctor and Patient. Judson Press, Valley Forge, Pa., 1977, pp 9–11.
2. Hardwig, J: Spirited Issues at the End of Life: A Call for Discussion. Hastings Center Report, 30(2), March–April 2000, pp 28–30.
3. Annas, GJ, Glantz, LH, and Katz, BF: The Rights of Doctors, Nurses and Allied Health Professionals. Avon Books, New York, 1981, p 228.
4. Munson, R: Intervention and Reflection: Basic Issues in Medical Ethics. Wadsworth, Belmont, Calif., 1992, p 147.

WEB RESOURCES

- ▲ Compassion and Choice. www.compassionandchoice.org
- ▲ Death with Dignity National Center. www.dwd.org
- ▲ National Hospice and Palliative Care Organization. www.nhpco.org
- ▲ World Federation of Right to Die. www.worldrtd.net

CHAPTER 16

Dying and Death

" *Death is not the greatest loss in life.
The greatest loss is what dies inside us while
we live.* "

Norman Cousins

LEARNING OBJECTIVES

Upon successful completion of this chapter, you will be able to:

1. Define key terms.
2. List at least eight generalizations about living with dying.
3. Compare short-term and long-term suffering.
4. Describe the importance of medications for dying clients.
5. Identify and explain at least five psychological aspects affecting dying clients.
6. Identify and explain at least five physiological aspects affecting dying clients.
7. Discuss the stages of dying as defined by Kübler-Ross.
8. Describe the services of hospice for dying clients.
9. Differentiate between active euthanasia and physician-assisted suicide.
10. Discuss the Uniform Anatomical Gift Act.
11. Describe an autopsy and who may authorize one.
12. Explain the role of physicians and health professionals in dying and death.

Vignette: What now?

Keith Nelson, aged 87, wakes in the middle of the night. The pain is sudden; it is over before he hit the floor. His life is gone. His wife of 62 years is asleep in the other bedroom. She finds her husband on the floor the next morning. She does not understand. The confusion she experiences in a brain diminished by early stages of Alzheimer's frightens her. Her only child, a daughter, lives in another state, but Mrs. Nelson does not remember the autodial number on the phone to call her daughter. She cannot remember 911. She dresses and puts on her makeup. Then she remembers that a police officer lives across the street. She stumbles across the street, rings the bell, and tells the sheriff, "I have trouble at home."

Death is the final stage of life. Dying is a process or a preparation for the final conclusion—death. For some, *dead* is a four-letter word not to be discussed; to others, the word represents an unpleasant reality difficult to think about or plan for. Some handle the concept realistically and well. In many respects, the way people face their dying or their death may be determined by how they live.

Most health professionals will work with clients who die and will respond to their surviving loved ones. How health professionals face this process may also be determined, in part, by how they face their own life and their own death. With the added knowledge from this chapter on dying and death, health care professionals can be better prepared to work with clients and their families during the dying-and-death process. Caring, understanding, and compassion are essential ingredients.

Living with Dying

Dying is a personal event. No two people die alike. Some die very quickly whereas others have time to plan for their deaths. Most hope for an easy death. To attempt to identify particular models for the "best" way to die is fruitless. None exists. Each person is unique, and the life experiences brought to the situation are varied. However, some helpful generalizations can be made.

1. The way people live is often mirrored in the way they die.
2. People with useful support systems, such as friends, family, and faith in life, may find this support helpful in dying.
3. Experiencing the death of someone close brings the reality of dying more into focus.
4. Intellectual preparation for dying, such as writing a will, an obituary, or planning a funeral may ease the fear of death.
5. Relationships with families and friends change.
6. Basic personalities usually remain unchanged, but moods may vary radically.
7. Personal goals are reevaluated.
8. Pain, suffering, and dependence are feared most by the dying.
9. Dying is not a casual experience.
10. The age of dying persons in part determines their reaction to death.
11. Persons who experience chronic disease or disability face their immortality more acutely than others.
12. Cultural mores influence attitudes toward death.

Suffering in Dying

Generally, everyone says they would prefer dying peacefully in their sleep or dying suddenly without warning or pain. In truth, most of us will lose our lives more gradually. Old age, debility, even senility may creep in before we realize that we have lost much of what we valued in our faculties. We may be diagnosed with a life-threatening illness that we believe will cause our death. Some will suffer in pain and agony. Some will be the object of medical experimentation and technology. It is this fear of suffering, the fear of dependence, the fear of loss of control, the fear of leaving loved ones, and the fear of pain that scares us most about death.

Short-term suffering presents a set of problems different from those of long-term suffering. This can best be seen in the following situations:

IN THE NEWS

A Harvard Medical School study states that elderly couples often seem to share times of death, sometimes the same day, week, month, or year. Close deaths of spouses may not be coincidental. Causes of close deaths of the elderly include severe distress due to the death or illness of a spouse, environment and habits that the couples share, and the fact that couples tend to pair with people who are most like themselves. The more the disease impairs the physical and mental functioning, the more harm it does to the health of the spouse. The remaining spouse is more at risk immediately after the spouse is hospitalized or dies.

Example 1

   A 45-year-old teacher learned in June that chronic myelocytic leukemia accompanied by blastic transformation was destroying his body. The prognosis was poor. Hospitalization and chemotherapy followed, with severe side effects and pain. He died 2 months later, never returning home.

Example 2

   A 50-year-old electrician was diagnosed as having cancer of the colon. Surgery followed, and a permanent colostomy was established. Postoperatively, the client did well and later returned to work part-time. Within a year, cancer metastasized and complications resulted. Consultation with specialists recommended only symptomatic treatment. Her pain required massive doses of analgesics to keep her comfortable for the remaining 6 months. The electrician was unable to return to work but remained home until about 6 weeks before death, when she was again hospitalized.

In a comparison of these two examples, time, costs, and dependency are three variables to consider. Obviously, the time of pain and suffering was longer for the electrician than for the teacher. The severity, however, cannot be compared. Overall costs are far greater for the electrician than the teacher, but nothing is known of insurance coverage or family resources. Either situation could be a financial burden on survivors. Dependency of these clients on their friends and family is somewhat different. The teacher had to depend on someone to take care of any personal matters, which might include job, children, and finances, for approximately 2 months. The electrician, however, was dependent on family for physical and nursing care in the home. She also needed someone to take care of personal matters from diagnosis to death, approximately 18 months.

   Even the length of time is difficult to establish. Time is relative; that is, 2 months and 18 months may both be considered short term when compared with an individual in a state of semiconsciousness for 4 or 5 years.

Use of Medications

Medications are used by the suffering when dying in both the hospital and at home. The greatest difficulty with medications arises in long-term suffering. Medications are given for many reasons, including analgesics for pain, sedatives for sleep, and specific medications for the particular disease condition. Antidepressants and tranquilizers also may be prescribed. Medications are to be respected for their intended action and the client's needs.

   Problems arise when family members, friends, and even health professionals circumvent or question the physician's orders for medications. This is often disastrous for the client. All persons close to the client ought to understand the physician's orders and the use of the pre-scribed medications. Family members should know the reasoning of the physician so that any questions arising are not misunderstood. For example, imagine the fear a loved one feels when the pharmacist says, "Do you know this is a near-lethal dose?" Unless the loved one knows that this amount is needed to keep the pain level of the client bearable, the loved one may withhold the medication and even begin to distrust the physician. Family members need to understand that medications may be given in different dosages, frequencies, and combina-tions for one dying client than for another. Age, weight, illness (whether chronic or acute), and the client's threshold for pain all influence a physician's choice of analgesics.

Sometimes physicians and health professionals are reluctant to prescribe or administer medications even though they are within the approved dosage range. In fact, in some cases health professionals will administer less than the prescribed dose because they believe what was prescribed was too much. Some may fear the client will become addicted. Phy-sicians may see opioid orders or prescriptions as crimes, not as treatment issues. They fear investigation. The client or family may want to use less than the amount prescribed because they believe it is too much. Clients may wait too long to ask for pain medica-tion, thinking they "can handle it." All have the potential of working against the clients' comfort.

▲ CRITICAL THINKING EXERCISE

If you knew you were going to die tomorrow, how differently would you live your life? Who will you make sure to talk with? Who will you write, call, or email? What regrets, if any, do you have?

Psychological Aspects of Dying

Dying clients differ in their psychological experiences. Although basic personalities remain the same, changes occur. A person normally calm and loving may have periods of violence and hostility. A happy person may become severely depressed. In fact, a person who is nearly comatose or close to death may be unaware of his or her responses to questions or be unable to make any decisions. An individual who usually is able to accept medical facts may totally deny a life-threatening illness.

Relationships may change. Some individuals are incapable of continuing a close relation-ship with a person who is dying. Closest friends may become aloof and distant. Some may fear touching or caressing the dying person. The dying person may reject any close contact or relationships. The following quotation, words from a dying person, illustrates this contro-versy: "I am not sure why, but I want to accept, and end up rejecting; I am willing to surren-der, but more often seek to control."[1] The opposite may also be true. A stronger bond of friendship can develop, and new friendships will be made, possibly from individuals in simi-lar circumstances. Broken relationships may be healed.

Relationships are important and should be encouraged. They provide strength and support that may not be available through any other source. The depth of relationships during this time and the degree of acceptance by dying clients may depend on their self-image. When a person is ill, is in pain, lives in a deteriorating body, and possibly is unable to perform the activities of daily living, self-image is fragile. When self-image is lacking, hope is lost; dying clients feel useless, may think they are burdens, and will have difficulties accepting help. The psychological effect of a poor self-image may even hasten death.

Dying clients may not be physically able to continue working. If they are sole wage earn-ers, this may present a financial crisis, especially if the unemployed period extends for a long time. Unemployed clients may be bored, feel useless, and worry, and their self-image suffers. For example, dying clients may worry that they are not fulfilling their usual role in the family and worry about their lack of control.

Personal goals for the dying person are altered or may even become nonexistent. Goals such as seeing a child graduate or a grandchild born may be seen as unrealistic to the dying because of limited time. The dying person either gives up or strives to live until a certain event takes place. The total loss of personal goals, no matter how insignificant they may appear, can be devastating to the dying and to persons caring for them. Goals may be different for the dying than for family members. Indecision is often a psychological dilemma accompanying the lack of personal goals. People close to the dying commonly recommend goals and help in the decision-making process. This must be done sensitively and realistically.

Communication may become difficult. Aside from any physiological problems precluding speech or communication, what dying clients are unable to understand or hear may depend on what they choose to hear or are ready to understand. Communication may be complicated further if the client's condition has not been honestly addressed. Of course, the opposite may be true. Some dying clients express the ability to communicate with greater depth because of the urgency of their circumstances.

Many communication difficulties center on the question of whether dying clients should be told of their terminal condition. How much information should they be given? Some people believe that all clients need to be told the medical facts by physicians and treated openly and honestly by all health professionals. They believe informed clients are better able to face death and are less afraid of the truth than are many health professionals. Other people believe no clients should be told they are dying, or that only those clients who give some verbal or nonverbal indication that they want to know should be told.

In some cultures, only family members and not the client are told of impending death. Only clients who can handle the truth should be told. Some clients may refuse to set goals, give up hope, and wait impatiently for death.

Fear is often a traumatic psychological aspect of dying. There is fear of pain, fear of long suffering, fear of losing independence, fear of financial ruin, and fear of death itself. The client's fears ought to be recognized and alleviated, if possible. To recognize these fears requires active and passive listening on the part of all people close to the dying individual and a willingness on the part of this individual to express those fears.

Much fear can be lessened if people close to the dying anticipate the fear and provide possible solutions and appropriate resources. Outside help may be sought, if necessary. Social workers, public health nurses, home health aides, clergy, and other health professionals can be valuable resources. Clients' fear should be taken seriously, and reference to their supposed unimportance should be avoided.

The psychological aspects of death are difficult for family, physicians, and health professionals because they may not be tangible. They generally are less understood than the physiological aspects of death and are often left to laypersons rather than professionals. To care for the physical and ignore the psychological is to treat only half the client.

▲ CRITICAL THINKING EXERCISE

In the Vignette at the beginning of the chapter, are there any end-of-life decisions that might have prevented the trauma Beulah must have felt when finding her husband dead? What actions would the sheriff need to take? Would an investigation need to be held?

Physiological Aspects of Dying

Medicine has numerous treatments for some of the physiological problems of suffering and pain experienced in the dying process. Sometimes the treatments are sufficient; at other times, they barely address the problem. Untreated or undiagnosed physiological problems may cause or enhance psychological difficulties for dying clients.

Separating the psychological from the physiological is difficult. For example, pain and suffering, if untreated by therapy or medicinal means, may prove to be a psychological barrier for clients, their families, and health professionals.

Loss of communication skills, such as in the aphasic client or in the comatose client, may be frustrating and unbearable. If clients are indecisive or suffer from dementia because of physiological changes, they may not be able to participate in the decision-making process of their life-threatening illness. Family members may need to assume greater roles in talking for clients and making decisions.

Other common physiological problems encountered include loss of bodily functions; inability to move or ambulate; inability to eat or drink; and inability to tolerate medications, treatments, light, or sound. In the hospital setting, these symptoms may be treated without much difficulty. However, if clients choose to die at home, professional help or training may prove valuable. If clients become severely disabled physically, they may be reluctant to go anywhere, even to the ambulatory health care setting. Family members may become exhausted caring for their loved ones or be unable to administer some of their treatments. The more severe these physiological problems, the more difficult daily existence becomes.

Physiological difficulties may hinder sexual identity and involvement. The expression of sexuality may be altered. The physiological and psychological aspects of sexuality are so intertwined that cause and effect are difficult to determine. It may be difficult or impossible to have sexual intercourse; however, there are many other ways to express love and caring or to relieve sexual tension. A discussion of the expression of sexuality and related client problems needs to be initiated with the client and partner.

Physiological and psychological problems are to be anticipated, diagnosed, and treated as much as possible. Treating the physiological and psychological aspects of clients enables total client care.

Stages of Grief

Elisabeth Kübler-Ross defines five stages of grief or responses to dying as follows. There is no set period for any one stage, nor will every dying person go through every stage. Some believe that no real grief work begins until you have been through all five stages. Some may stay in denial until death; others may manage denial and bargaining and stumble in depression. Still others may move back and forth from one stage to another. Some may move through some or all of the stages several times. There is no set or acceptable pattern. Each dying client is an individual, as are family members. However, the stages do offer information on how to relate to clients and their families, who will experience similar stages.

 Elisabeth Kübler-Ross defines five stages of dying and death:

1. Denial
2. Anger
3. Bargaining
4. Depression
5. Acceptance

Denial

Clients may deny their life-threatening or terminal illness or go through periods of disbelief. Sometimes it is a result of shock when they are first told. Clients commonly say, "This is not happening to me" or "I'll go to another physician to see what's wrong." Denial generally is a temporary defense and offers therapeutic meaning to clients.

Health professionals should listen to clients during this stage. Trying to contradict clients or force them to believe what is happening to them will be to no avail. Encourage clients to talk about death. Listen, listen, and listen.

Anger

Clients suddenly realize "It is me. This is happening to me. Why me?" They may become "problem clients" and are envious and resentful. Anger may be dispersed in all directions, at people and toward the environment. Rage and temper tantrums can occur. Professionals and family members need to be understanding no matter how angry the client becomes. Listening to clients is important to allow them to vent their own feelings.

Bargaining

During this stage, clients try to make deals with physicians, God or higher being, or family, usually for more time or for a period of comfort without pain. Clients tend to be more cooperative and congenial. Common responses include the following: "Please let me see my homeland again." "I'll be so good, if I can just have 3 pain-free hours." "Dear God, I'll never … if you make me well." Health professionals can listen to dying clients' requests but not become a party to the bargain. Some bargaining may be associated with guilt, and any indication of this should be mentioned to the physician. Bargaining can have a positive effect. It may give the client the hope and stamina to reach a desired goal. It is OK to mourn and cry. Allow for silences.

Depression

The dying client's body is deteriorating, sometimes rapidly; financial burdens are likely increasing; pain is unbearable; and relationships are severed. All can lead to depression. The dying are losing everything and everyone they love. Dying may be a time of tears, and crying may allow relief. Professionals who are happy, loud, and reassuring will not provide much help to depressed clients. Clients may need to express their sorrow to someone or merely have someone close. They may have little need for words at this stage. Simple tasks may be impossible. Helplessness is real.

Acceptance

The final but perhaps not lasting stage is when clients are accepting of their fate. They usually are tired, weak, and able to sleep. They are not necessarily happy, but rather at peace. Professionals will be aware that clients may prefer to be left alone and not bothered with world events or family problems. Family members usually require more help, understanding, and support than clients in this stage. Touching and the use of silence may prove helpful.

▲ CRITICAL THINKING EXERCISE

Relate the five stages identified by Kübler-Ross to any death or grieving experience you have had. Did you pass through all the stages? What was/is most difficult for you?

Throughout the experience of loss, there will come a time when friends and neighbors stop calling, "closure" has occurred by the dying person and everything is slowly getting back to normal. Some say this is when the real grief work begins. A common definition of grief work is summarized by the acronym TEAR.

T = To accept the reality of the loss
E = Experience the pain of the loss
A = Adjust to the environment of what was lost
R = Reinvest in the new reality

Hospice

Dictionaries define the term hospice as "lodging for travelers or young persons, especially when maintained by a religious order." The term later was used to describe lodging for dying clients. The first such hospice, Saint Christopher's, was formed by Cecily Saunders in London in 1965. Since then, the hospice concept has expanded throughout the United States.

Hospice provides care for the terminally ill at home, in a hospital, in a skilled nursing home, or in a special hospice facility. The main objective of care is to make clients comfortable, "at home," and close to family. Treatments such as cardiopulmonary resuscitation, intravenous therapy, nasogastric tubes, and antibiotics are discouraged. Treatments are given in light of the client's personal and social circumstances.

The hospice staff attempts to create a positive atmosphere. Death is seen as "all right." A balance is kept between human needs and medical needs. Children are encouraged to be in the hospice as a reminder that life is an ongoing process. Clients might share a cup of tea with staff and each other rather than receiving an intravenous solution during their last hours.

An advantage hospice offers is staff members who are experienced and want to care for the dying. Its services are provided only to the dying, and death is managed with dignity. The expense is generally less than acute care costs, and may be covered by insurance. In a special hospice facility, the dying client is not isolated behind curtains but rather is surrounded by others. An empty bed remains empty for at least 24 hours to allow adjustment by everyone. In addition, survivors are helped to deal with the death. If the hospice care is at home, clients are in familiar surroundings, may have their favorite foods, and are close to loved ones.

The hospice does have disadvantages. One problem is whether family members, with a hospice's help, can handle the care at home. It may be too much, physically and emotionally. Also, what about dying clients? Are they comfortable with the kind of care they receive in the hospice? Do they need or want more? Are they comfortable dealing with death? We may be conditioned to expect dying clients to be in hospitals, not homes.

Physician-Assisted Death

Questions arise about whether physician-assisted death or euthanasia should be endorsed. Are the two similar, or are they different enough that the arguments for one do not apply to the other? It is physician-assisted suicide when the physician provides a client with a lethal dose of medication so that the client can self-administer the medication; it is active euthanasia when a physician administers a lethal dose to the client. In case of either physician-assisted death or euthanasia, the physician is active and involved; however, in both cases the client decides whether to ask for the medication. The client makes the choices in dying. In physician-assisted death, the client acts last, whereas in active euthanasia, the physician acts last.

Just as California and Washington were forerunners with their living wills and natural death laws, they were forerunners in seeking legislation that would give people the option to seek "aid in dying from physicians to end life in a dignified, painless and humane manner." Such proposed laws are much broader in their scope than any living will or physicians' directive. To date neither state has passed physician-assisted suicide laws.

In 1994, Oregon passed the Death with Dignity measure that was later challenged by the courts. In 1997, the act was reaffirmed by the Oregon voters. The measure is the nation's first and, to date, the only state to allow a physician to prescribe a lethal dose of medication when asked by a terminally ill client. The four safeguards for this measure are as follows: (1) the attending physician must truly convey informed consent, which must include all feasible opportunities such as pain management, hospice, and palliative care. (2) The attending physician's diagnosis and prognosis must be confirmed by a consulting physician. The latter physician must verify that the client has made a voluntary and informed decision. (3) If either physician thinks the client might have depression that might impair judgment, a counseling session must be attended. (4) The client making the request must do so both orally and in writing. The law details specific time lines and a waiting period for the client before receiving the lethal medication. The request must be witnessed by at least two people who can verify the client's capacity to make a decision and that the decision is voluntary. Obviously, the measure poses valid concerns, but it is a testimony to the growing desire to have increased legal protection for options in dying.

Once the Oregon Death with Dignity Act was reaffirmed in 1997 by Oregon voters, 16 people were assisted in suicide in 1998. Most recent statistics, available at this writing, indicate 33 individuals in 2004 and 35 in 2005. The median age of the individuals was 64 to 70 years. The majority of these individuals had end-stage cancer. Chronic lung disease was also common. The majority were in hospice before death.

In fall 2001, U.S. Attorney General Ashcroft determined that the government would step in to revoke the licenses of any physician who prescribed controlled substances to clients seeking physician-assisted death in Oregon. By a 6-to-3 vote the U. S. Supreme Court ruled that Ashcroft exceeded his authority when he tried to block the Oregon law to help terminally ill clients die. The Supreme Court decision opens the door for other states to legalize physician-assisted death. Some predict that California and Vermont will be the next states to pass similar legislation.

In 1997, the U.S. Senate passed a bill barring the federal government from financing physician-assisted death. The vote was 99 to 0. The same measure previously cleared the House of Representatives by a vote of 398 to 16. Medicare and Medicaid are prohibited from funding physician-assisted death. In June 1997, all nine Supreme Court justices refused to accept the fact that assisted death was a fundamental liberty for the terminally ill.

Legislation on physician-assisted death continues to be controversial, contradictory, confusing, and as emotional as legalization of abortion has been in the United States. Some questions to ponder on the subject include the following: Will potentially lethal medications be restricted? How accurate can the prediction of death within 6 months be? Will a working definition of "terminal" be relaxed? Can physicians recognize depression or the inability of a client to make such a choice? What happens to the client who asks for a lethal medication but is unable to administer it? Are that person's rights less than those of the person who is able to administer the dose?

▲ CRITICAL THINKING EXERCISE

The U.S. Supreme Court ruled on Washington state's and New York state's assisted-death laws. They rejected the notion that assisted death is a fundamental liberty. The nation's newspapers revealed that one justice's wife died of cancer; another justice is a cancer survivor, and a third justice's spouse works with cancer clients. Discuss.

IN THE NEWS

A male nurse, who worked in a clinic in Bavaria, Germany, has admitted to "ending the lives" of 12 of the 29 patients he is accused of killing. He said he carried out acts of compassion when he administered lethal injections to his patients. When police searched his home, they found enough unsealed vials to kill ten people. Relatives of the deceased patients say some who died were not even in his care and some were not seriously ill.

A doctor and two nurses are accused of killing four patients in the aftermath of Hurricane Katrina in a New Orleans, Louisiana hospital. The patients, among the sickest in the city, could not be evacuated. After Katrina, the hospital conditions were deplorable. The accused used lethal injections of morphine and a sedative that stop the heart and lungs. The attorney general says, "This is not euthanasia. This is homicide." Or is it compassion in dying or assisted death?

Uniform Anatomical Gift Act

The legal definition of death is particularly important in the area of organ transplants. All 50 states have some form of the Uniform Anatomical Gift Act. Persons 18 years or older and of sound mind may make a gift of all or any part of their body to the following persons for the following purposes:

1. To any hospital, surgeon, or physician for medical or dental education, research, advancement of medical or dental science, therapy, or transplantation
2. To any accredited medical or dental school, college, or university for education, research, advancement of medical or dental science, or therapy
3. To any organ bank or storage facility, for medical or dental education, research, advancement of medical or dental science, therapy, or transplantation
4. To any specified individual for therapy or transplantation needed by him or her

The gift may be made by a provision in a will or by signing, in the presence of two witnesses, a card. The card is generally carried with the person at all times. The latter method is the best because the living will may not be readily available until it is too late for donation of organs or tissues. Donated organs include heart, lung, kidney, pancreas, liver, and intestine; tissue includes eyes, skin, bone, heart valves, veins, and tendons. There is no cost to the donors or their families. Generally, there is no cost for later cremation or burial of the body parts. In Pennsylvania, organ donors and their families may receive a fee for organ donation through a program administered by the state Department of Health.

 It is illegal to sell body parts in this country; however, the practice is common in developing countries. It is becoming increasingly popular to find compatible

---

IN THE NEWS

Mount Sinai Hospital in Manhattan does more living donors for liver transplants than any other hospital in the United States, but an incident occurred that ethicists and surgeons have dreaded since the use of live donors for transplants. A 57-year-old healthy man donated part of his liver to his brother and the donor died three days later. The recipient lived. Neither the hospital nor the widow would comment. In a liver transplant, surgeons remove the right lobe of the donor's liver and the pieces in both donor and recipient grow back to full size in about a month, if all goes well. The live donor faces all the risks of surgery. What are the benefits of the donor?

donors for transplant organs on the Internet. Many clients needing a transplant organ are setting up websites to tell their life stories and make electronic pleas in chat rooms for willing donors. One such example reports of a 32-year-old man suffering with liver cancer who took out newspaper ads, set up a toll-free number, and bought space on two billboards along busy highways to appeal for a liver donor. In just a few months, he was rewarded with a liver from a deceased donor. Another example tells of an individual on a waiting list for a kidney for 5 years who paid monthly fees to have his profile posted on www.matchingdonors.com. He received 500 offers for a donation, found a match, and is expected to pay his donor $5,000 in transportation costs and other expenses incurred. About 90,000 Americans are on lists for organs, mostly kidneys and livers. Many will die waiting. Because less than 20% of American adults are registered organ donors, and only 50% of families agree to donate organs of their deceased loved ones when asked, bartering for organs will continue.

Persons may place conditions on their organ donation. If a relative opposes the donation, most physicians and hospitals would not insist on the transplant. Donors are carefully screened before their body parts are used. The physician and hospital may be found negligent, so they must have strict standards for donor screening.

 Cultural differences exist, as well as religious differences, in cases of organ and tissue donation. For example, the Hmong immigrants from Southeast Asia may believe that organ donation prevents the person from experiencing reincarnation; for this reason, the Hmong also resist autopsies. Many Native Americans oppose organ donation because of their enormous reverence for the body that is considered both the residence and the manifestation of a person's essence. Health care professionals will want to be sensitive to, understand, and appreciate cultural preferences.

Autopsy

An autopsy is an examination of a dead body to determine the cause of death. Statutes generally state who can authorize an autopsy and under what circumstances. Coroners or medical examiners may give such authorization. Others include, in order of priority:

🔑 Priority Authorization for Autopsy

1. The surviving spouse
2. Any child of the deceased who is 18 years of age or older
3. Any one of the parents of the deceased
4. Any adult sibling of the deceased

Autopsies may be complete or partial. In other words, a pathologist may perform an autopsy on the entire body and examine every part and organ or do an autopsy only of the thoracic cavity or the brain. The extremities rarely are involved unless indicated by trauma, prior surgical procedure, or vessel involvement. No parts of the body can be retained for any reason without consent from the family. If the autopsy is done properly and in a professional manner, the body can be viewed by survivors or at a death ritual.

Some circumstances require an autopsy to investigate the cause of a suspicious death. Autopsies also offer valuable information for medical science and research. Survivors need to understand that knowledge gained from an autopsy may prevent another person from suffering similar circumstances. Refer to Chapter 6 for further information on autopsy.

The Role of Health Professionals

Clients with life-threatening or terminal illnesses have special needs. Their reactions in the dying process are expressed in their various stages or responses. Regardless of how they present themselves, health professionals need to assess where clients are and react openly to them.

One of the best ways to begin interacting with the dying client is to take a good, hard look at your own attitudes toward pain, suffering, and dying. How can you be especially sensitive to these clients without being obvious? Will you be able to respond to the client's total needs rather than merely the client's medical needs? Can you be comfortable when clients cry, when clients laugh, when they joke about their condition?

Health care professionals need to be able to talk without fear or anxiety as they provide information, and they must be able to listen to dying clients. For example, a health care employee may be asked, "Will I get addicted to these pain pills?" If the employee's thoughts are, "The doctor never should have given you anything so powerful," this attitude will be sensed by the client.

Dying clients may exhibit negative or distasteful behaviors in the health care setting. How will you handle it? Will you take it personally? React negatively? Ignore it? Clients may ask questions with hidden meanings or be truly blunt. Are you aware of nonverbal clues from clients? How will you react? What if you do not know any answers?

Dying clients may develop gross physical deformities or radically altered physical appearances. Will you be able to manage? If so, how? Family and friends also will require your attention. What will you do when you reach the end of your rope or become too emotionally involved? Client referrals may be made to counselors, clergy, attorneys, social workers, and hospice organizations. Do not fool yourself that you can be all things to all people. Health professionals should feel free to refer.

After the client has died, physicians and employees will turn their focus to the survivors. In telling survivors of the death, be honest and caring. It is a sorrowful and painful time for survivors, and they will need your utmost attention. Try to provide whatever support they need and remain with them until some family or close friends can come.

During the grieving process, survivors may call or come to the ambulatory health care setting for information or assistance. If you are unable to answer their questions or meet their needs, refer them to someone who can. Funeral directors and the clergy offer valuable help in planning the funeral or death ritual, answering questions about the human remains, and helping survivors through the grieving process. Organizations such as Compassionate Friends (parents and families who have lost a child) and groups for widows or widowers can be recommended, if appropriate.

Children and death pose sensitive situations. The death of a child is a profound emotional experience for everyone, especially family. Explaining death to a child is also difficult. The age and maturity of children are to be considered. Children deserve the same honesty as an adult and need to be told that sorrow is acceptable and crying is okay. Reassure children that death is in no way their fault. Using a phrase such as "God took your daddy away" may cause the child to blame God. Follow the lead of children in their questions, and tell children you do not have all the answers. Memories should be cherished and encouraged. Children require the same ritual and sorrow that other family members do, but do not force them to attend a funeral if they do not want to.

Summary

Volumes have been written in the past decade on the subject of dying and death. The information in this chapter merely highlights the areas that seem most appropriate for health professionals who play a key role in educating clients and their families by answering questions, making referrals to appropriate resources, and carrying brochures and information that pertain to dying and death issues.

QUESTIONS FOR REVIEW

1. Explain the use of medications with the dying client.

_____

_____

2. List the psychological aspects of dying.

_____

_____

3. List the physiological aspects of dying.

_____

_____

4. Identify the stages of grief.

_____

_____

5. Describe the services of hospice.

_____

_____

6. List the latest legislation on physician-assisted death.

_____

_____

7. Describe the purpose of the Uniform Anatomical Gift.

_____

_____

8. Define autopsy.

_____

_____

CLASSROOM QUESTIONS

1. Are there any generalizations on death that you might add to the authors'? Any you might delete? Which ones most likely would describe you?

2. Describe some problems faced by family members involved with a long-term illness.

3. Does the allocation of scarce medical resources influence the care given to someone who is dying?

4. List Kübler-Ross's five stages of dying and grief and give an example of each that you have experienced.

5. A client leaves the ambulatory health care setting and says to the receptionist, "I know I am dying. You people are lying to me." What is your response?

6. Would you prefer to die in a hospice or a hospital? Justify your answer.

7. Enter into a discussion wherein you identify and discuss reasons why physician-assisted death meets with so much controversy. Do you agree or disagree?

8. Would you donate your organs or tissues? If so, which ones? If not, explain.

9. Under what circumstances might physicians decide not to tell clients they are dying?

10. What considerations are taken into account when telling a child about death?

11. Why might an autopsy be helpful? Why might one be refused?

12. What have you done to prepare for your own death? Do you have a will? Have you planned for your family? Have you made any decisions that should be shared with legal counsel or physicians?

13. Refer to Ted's case in Chapter 15. Could Ted's inability to respond to the nephrologist's question about dialysis imply that he had changed his mind regarding heroic measures? Who would be the best person to determine this?

REFERENCES

1. Smith, JK: Free Fall. Judson, Valley Forge, Pa., 1975, p 7.

WEB RESOURCES

▲ American Academy of Child and Adolescent Psychiatry, Children and Grief. www.aacap.org
▲ American Association of Retired People (AARP). Grief and Loss. www.aarp.org
▲ Boston.com. Doctor-assisted suicide gains ground; Supreme Court rejects bid to block Oregon Law. www.boston.com
▲ Counseling for Loss and Life Changes. Beware of the 5 Stages of "Grief." www.counselingforloss.com/article8.htm
▲ Donate Life. http://www.organdonor.gov
▲ eMedicine Consumer Health. Grief and Bereavement. www.emedicine.com
▲ Living Bank, www.livingbank.org
▲ National Mental Health Association. Coping with Loss, Bereavement and Grief. www.nmha.org
▲ State of Oregon, Death with Dignity Act. www.oregon.gov/DHS
▲ State of Pennsylvania, Department of Health. www.dsf.health.state.pa.us/health

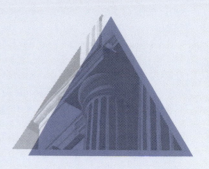

Have a Care!

Carol's Note

I have been a colleague, friend, confidant, and certainly receiver of Marti Lewis's resilience throughout the many years of our friendship. Never once have I heard or seen her complain, ask "Why me?" or come close to giving up.

When Marti and I wrote the first edition of this text, she would not talk much about her illness. "Have a Care" came about because Marti's story told more poignantly about the importance of being sensitive and compassionate toward your clients than anything we could possibly have written without it.

After you read her story, I think you'll understand why.

Marti's Story

It's early December, many years ago. I hurt. I can't function at home. I can't function at work. The pain in my back is so bad I can't lift my 5-month-old infant. It hurts to shower and turn the steering wheel of the car. I have to go to bed before my husband and then I can't move. The spasms are terrifying. They wake me.

I am so tired. I have no energy. I'm not really afraid. I trust my doctor. I know he'll find out what is wrong, fix it, and I'll be back to normal. I'm taking time from work to go to my doctor's office. It is inconvenient, but I can do it. No one will do my job while I'm gone; it will wait for my return. I expect action today, though. I don't want sympathy.

I'm glad I don't have to wait long in the clinic. The pain is a little less; the psychological release from knowing I'll soon be better is addicting. But I put up a front, too. I can't cry or tell the doctor how bad the pain really is. The assistant's greeting is cheerful, but I could use some help with my clothes. I can hardly get them off. The bra is terrible, and the pantyhose are worse.

My physician is quiet, professional, and concerned. I feel better just seeing him. His smile is warm. I can tell he cares. The examination is not too difficult. He finally says, "It looks serious. We have to run a lot of tests. It is going to take time to get to the bottom of this." Laboratory tests and x-rays are ordered. Any physical activity is allowed until it causes pain. I don't tell him how hard that will be. He tells me to bring my husband with me the next visit. I'm instructed to get dressed and go to the laboratory. The awful bra and pantyhose again, and it hurts to tie my shoes.

The atmosphere is sterile in the laboratory—cool and too professional. My mind is racing while I wait. I'm in torment. "What is it? What about my baby? Will I be able to take care of her? I've waited 36 years for her. Am I going to be a burden?"

The laboratory technician withdraws the blood, and I give the laboratory a urine specimen. The awful pantyhose again! "Collect a 24-hour urine." They hand me this weird, antifreeze-like container with an opening like a vinegar bottle. It is white and has large black letters: "For 24-Hour Urine Only." I also am told to collect some feces. I'm handed three unfolded cardboard containers and some tiny spatulas. No instructions.

As I leave, I wonder, how long do I wait? When will I know? I'm exhausted. I want to get home and see my husband. I need to talk to someone. Oh, the pain is bad. I hurt.

A telephone call a week later from my physician tells me the progress of the tests, but no indication of a diagnosis. His conversation is very general.

Christmas is a blur. There is no change in my condition. Questions from family and friends are no help. They don't understand. Neither do I. I hide my true feelings.

I'm back in the doctor's office a few weeks later with my husband. He had to take time from work. The receptionist seems surprised that my husband is with me. I wonder if she thinks I can't handle this. Well, I can't!

The consultation is hard. My physician is open and honest—he tells us that a bone disease is rampant. It is a metabolic bone disorder. I hear him tell my husband that I can have no physical activity. I must take off work. I cannot drive. To fall would be disastrous. My bones are like a loaf of bread. "You know what a loaf of bread is like when it is smashed." I cannot lift anything, even my baby. I'm not supposed to bend over. My husband asks, "Should we have outside help come into the home?" The doctor says, "Yes." I immediately think about the cost. The doctor tells me what kind of medications I'll be taking. But the final blow is his words that something else is wrong. He hopes more tests will reveal what.

A month passes. I'm having such a hard time having someone do my work. A replacement is hired for my job. I don't ask for help easily. It is so hard to be inactive. I can't get my own groceries. I'm terrified of falling. I can't vacuum my floors. I can't lift my baby to change her. If she cries, I can't pick her up. Having someone else do the things I'm supposed to do is terrible. When no one is looking, I do lift her. I do carry her. And I do damage my body. This creates conflict with my husband. Life is not good.

During this time, there are more tests. More referrals. More doctors. I feel like a nothing. I feel inhuman. The worst tests are the small bowel biopsies. My physician tells me that they will put a tube in my mouth and pass it through to the small intestine. He says it is painless and won't take very long.

My husband takes me to the test and is told I'll be finished in about 1 hour. They will call him. In the examination room, I'm partially disrobed, and I put on a full-length gown that opens down the back. I can keep my slacks and shoes on. The gastroenterologist passes the tube through my mouth into my stomach. There is no pain, but it is awful. I gag over and over again. I must try not to. I tell myself to breathe slowly, to concentrate on not vomiting. When the gastroenterologist finishes, the LPN says, "Let's go to x-ray."

To my horror, she hands me a box of tissues and an emesis basin, drapes my coat over my shoulders, takes my elbow, and says, "Be careful not to fall." I bite on the tube in my mouth and try to stabilize it with my free hand as we walk through a large, crowded reception area, out the front door, and across two office parking lots covered with early morning frost. While I am still in disbelief, we walk into the lowest floor of a multiple-office building where the x-ray receptionist tells us the radiologist is still at the hospital making rounds. I snarl through my teeth, "Get that doctor here now."

In the x-ray waiting area, I sit for 30 minutes, still trying not to gag. The tears come, first haltingly, then freely. The saliva flows from my mouth and nose. I'm finally able to get a hold of myself. I stop crying. I don't want to ruin the test. Finally the doctor appears. He looks at me. In my revulsion at the situation and him, I whisper, "You son of a —!" His response is, "What's wrong with you?" How can I tell him? I still have the tube in my mouth. He checks the placement of the tube in the small intestine several different times. When he verifies that it is in place, he calls another LPN to take me back. Over the same route. I pray to God no one recognizes me. I am in a state of shock about my circumstances.

Upon returning, the biopsy is taken. The doctor pulls the tube. I sigh with relief. In a few minutes, he turns to me and says, "We didn't get it." The instrument to snatch a piece of the intestinal wall didn't grab properly. The same procedure must be done again. The tube goes back in, across the parking lots; check the tube, back across the parking lots. This time, the biopsy is successful.

This whole time my husband is trying to call the office and wondering what has happened. They tell him only that there is a problem. He is not allowed to speak to anyone else. Four-and-a-half hours later, they call to tell him I'm finished.

Ten years have passed. I'm now living with the metabolic bone disorder, which is somewhat improved. I have an intestinal malabsorption problem that is totally controlled by diet. My activities are somewhat limited. I cannot lift anything heavy or participate in any sport other than swimming, but I no longer need help at home. I must take a lot of medication, some of it is experimental, and I'm 4 inches shorter.

I have a hearing loss that requires the use of hearing aids. Speech sounds are distorted. Pain is always with me. I am afraid I will someday be confined to a wheelchair and fear that I might have to quit work. I wonder why my body has to be so "unusual."

On good days, I remind myself that I must live in the here and now. I continue my teaching with urgency. I am glad I can handle pain. I thank God daily for my coauthor, who brings out the best in me. (Someday I will be as short as she is.) I practice a healthful lifestyle and willingly share my sense of humor. I enjoy life to the very fullest. My family and friends give me strength. I've loved being an author of this book.

And now 28 years have gone by. It was beyond my wildest imagination during the writing of the first edition of this book in early 1980 what life would bring to me in the next 30 years—in fact, I doubted I'd still be alive, but I thank God I am. The challenges have been great. Never did I believe that I would:

▲ Be 5 inches shorter
▲ Still not be able to lift anything more than 5 pounds
▲ Experience such a severe hearing loss
▲ Know spinal pain so excruciating it strikes like lightning and steals my breath and grips me with fear
▲ Have no respite from exhaustive, ever present, night and day, throbbing pain
▲ Never have another piece of "real" berry pie or a chocolate chip cookie
▲ Sometimes wake up screaming, unable to move because of pinched nerves
▲ Fear that I might someday be paralyzed

▲ Yell and scream obscenities at God when I am most angry about my illness
▲ Become such an intimate friend of the 5 stages of grief

Yet, to tell you of my challenges and not my blessings would be a sham. I could not have believed that my blessings would be so bountiful and so rewarding. I have:

▲ An excellent and sensitive primary care physician, bone specialist, and gastroenterologist
▲ A husband who is a solid rock, my love, and thinks I can do no wrong—until I forget and lift more than 5 pounds
▲ A strong, competent, sensitive daughter who has finished graduate school and loves her job
▲ The authorship of two quite successful books of which I am very proud
▲ A true and transparent friend with whom I write and cavort
▲ Parents with whom I walked "through the valley of death" and learned so much
▲ A successful career in the medical assistant/nursing fields
▲ Retirement that is liberating beyond my belief
▲ A toy poodle named "Tiny" and a black cat "Sammy," that I get to love and spoil
▲ An incredible capacity for laughter and play
▲ Love of music and chocolate and more chocolate!

Carol and I share this story with you because we care. We hope that by sharing the story of my condition you'll be better able to share your own compassion. Remember to be loving, gracious, human, and able to put yourself in the place of your clients. Remember that the client is more than someone with an illness or injury. Clients are people with responsibilities, families, and personal and emotional needs.

I will be forever grateful to the health care professionals who have treated me with respect and compassion and forever curious about those who haven't. Please, throughout your career as a health care professional, do your clients and yourself a huge favor: *Have a care!*

Final Note from Carol

Marti has been more than my equal. She has seen me through a divorce and encouraged me when I dated and then remarried. She mentors and loves my daughters even as they have become mothers and counsels me when I need advice. She helped me work through my grief when my parents died within 15 months of each other. She comes when I call and makes no fuss when I carry the bags. She is still going when I am ready to drop, like the battery that keeps going and going and going.

Together now, we walk along the beach and river. Sometimes it is shallow, rocky, and hard. We wade in together, holding onto each other. Sometimes the river is deep, sweeps us off our feet, and we float freely in warmth and peace. Sometimes there are bends in the river, bends we can't see around, and it scares us. But we go on. We are reminded constantly (thank you, Judy Collins) that:

"In the valleys, we look for the mountains.
In the mountains, we've searched for the rivers.
There is nowhere to go. We are where we belong.
We can and do live the life we dreamed."

— Marti Lewis and Carol Tamparo

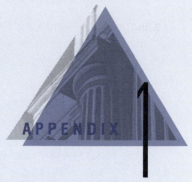

Codes of Ethics

1. **The Hippocratic Oath**
2. **American Association of Medical Assistants**
3. **Principles of Medical Ethics: American Medical Association**

The Hippocratic Oath[*]

I swear by Apollo Physician and Aslepius and Hygieia and Panaceia and all the gods and goddesses, making them my witnesses, that I will fulfil according to my ability and judgment this oath and this covenant:

To hold him who has taught me this art as equal to my parents and to live my life in partnership with him, and if he is in need of money to give him a share of mine, and to regard his offspring as equal to my brothers in male lineage and to teach them this art if they desire to learn it without fee and covenant; to give a share of precepts and oral instruction and all the other learning to my sons and to the sons of him who has instructed me and to pupils who have signed the covenant and have taken an oath according to the medical law, but to no one else.

I will apply dietetic measures for the benefit of the sick according to my ability and judgment; I will keep them from harm and injustice.

I will neither give a deadly drug to anybody if asked for it, nor will I make a suggestion to this effect. Similarly I will not give to a woman an abortive remedy. In purity and holiness I will guard my life and my art.

I will not use the knife, not even on sufferers from stone, but will withdraw in favor of such men as are engaged in this work.

Whatever houses I may visit, I will come for the benefit of the sick, remaining free of all intentional injustice, of all mischief and in particular of sexual relations with both female and male persons, be they free or slaves.

What I may see or hear in the course of the treatment or even outside of the treatment in regard to the life of men, which on no account one must spread abroad, I will keep to myself holding such things shameful to be spoken about.

[*]From Ludwig, E: The Hippocratic oath. In Oswei, T, and Temkin, CL (eds): Ancient Medicine. Johns Hopkins University Press, Baltimore, 1967, with permission.

If I fulfil this oath and do not violate it, may it be granted to me to enjoy life and art, being honored with fame among all men for all time to come; if I transgress it and swear falsely, may the opposite of all this be my lot.

American Association of Medical Assistants

The Code of Ethics of AAMA shall set forth principles of ethical and moral conduct as they relate to the medical profession and the particular practice of medical assisting.

Members of AAMA dedicated to the conscientious pursuit of their profession, and thus desiring to merit the high regard of the entire medical profession and the respect of the general public which they serve, do pledge themselves to strive always to:

A. Render service with full respect for the dignity of humanity;
B. Respect confidential information obtained through employment unless legally authorized or required by responsible performance of duty to divulge such information;
C. Uphold the honor and high principles of the profession and accept its disciplines;
D. Seek to continually improve the knowledge and skills of medical assistants for the benefit of patients and professional colleagues;
E. Participate in additional service activities aimed toward improving the health and well-being of the community.

Creed

I believe in the principles and purposes of the profession of medical assisting.
I endeavor to be more effective.
I aspire to render greater service.
I protect the confidence entrusted to me.
I am dedicated to the care and well-being of all people.
I am loyal to my employer.
I am true to the ethics of my profession.
I am strengthened by compassion, courage, and faith.

Principles of Medical Ethics: American Medical Association[†]

Preamble

The medical profession has long subscribed to a body of ethical statements developed primarily for the benefit of the patient. As a member of this profession, a physician must recognize responsibility to patients first and foremost, as well as to society, to other health professionals, and to self. The following Principles adopted by the American Medical Association are not laws, but standards of conduct that define the essentials of honorable behavior for the physician.

Principles of Medical Ethics

I. A physician shall be dedicated to providing competent medical care, with compassion and respect for human dignity and rights.

[†]From the American Medical Association, adopted by the American Medical Association's House of Delegates June 17, 2001. Reprinted with permission from American Medical Association, Code of Medical Ethics, Copyright 2000.

II. A physician shall uphold the standards of professionalism, be honest in all professional interactions, and strive to report physicians deficient in character or competence, or engaging in fraud or deception, to appropriate entities.

III. A physician shall respect the law and also recognize a responsibility to seek changes in those requirements which are contrary to the best interests of the patient.

IV. A physician shall respect the rights of patients, colleagues, and other health professionals, and shall safeguard patient confidences and privacy within the constraints of the law.

V. A physician shall continue to study, apply, and advance scientific knowledge, maintain a commitment to medical education, make relevant information available to patients, colleagues, and the public, obtain consultation, and use the talents of other health professionals when indicated.

VI. A physician shall, in the provision of appropriate patient care, except in emergencies, be free to choose whom to serve, with whom to associate, and the environment in which to provide medical care.

VII. A physician shall recognize a responsibility to participate in activities contributing to the improvement of the community and the betterment of public health.

VIII. A physician shall, while caring for a patient, regard responsibility to the patient as paramount.

IX. A physician shall support access to medical care for all people.

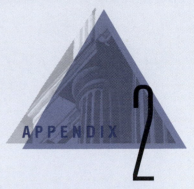

Sample Documents for Choices about Health Care, Life, and Death

INSTRUCTIONS
───────

PRINT THE DATE

PRINT YOUR NAME

WASHINGTON HEALTH CARE DIRECTIVE

Directive made this _____ day of _____, _____.
　　　　　　　　　　(date)　　　　　*(month)*　　　　　　*(year)*

I, _____,
　　　　　　　　　　　　　　　(name)

having the capacity to make health care decisions, willfully, and voluntarily make known my desire that my dying shall not be artificially prolonged under the circumstances set forth below, and do hereby declare that:

(a) If at any time I should be diagnosed in writing to be in a terminal condition by the attending physician, or in a permanent unconscious condition by two physicians, and where the application of life-sustaining treatment would serve only to artificially prolong the process of my dying, I direct that such treatment be withheld or withdrawn, and that I be permitted to die naturally. I understand by using this form that a terminal condition means an incurable and irreversible condition caused by injury, disease, or illness, that would within reasonable medical judgment cause death within a reasonable period of time in accordance with accepted medical standards, and where the application of life-sustaining treatment would serve only to prolong the process of dying. I further understand in using this form that a permanent unconscious condition means an incurable and irreversible condition in which I am medically assessed within reasonable medical judgment as having no reasonable probability of recovery from an irreversible coma or a persistent vegetative state.

(b) In the absence of my ability to give directions regarding the use of such life-sustaining treatment, it is my intention that this directive shall be honored by my family and physician(s) as the final expression of my legal right to refuse medical or surgical treatment and I accept the consequences of such refusal. If another person is appointed to make these decisions for me, whether through a durable power of attorney or otherwise, I request that the person be guided by this directive and any other clear expressions of my desires.

INDICATE YOUR WISHES ABOUT ARTIFICIAL FEEDING

© 2000
PARTNERSHIP FOR
CARING, INC.

(c) If I am diagnosed to be in a terminal condition or in a permanent unconscious condition (check one):
　❏ I DO want to have artificially provided nutrition and hydration.
　❏ I DO NOT want to have artificially provided nutrition and
　　　hydration.

WASHINGTON HEALTH CARE DIRECTIVE — PAGE 2 OF 2

ADD PERSONAL INSTRUCTIONS (IF ANY)

(d) If I have been diagnosed as pregnant and that diagnosis is known to my physician, this directive shall have no force or effect during the course of my pregnancy.

(e) I understand the full import of this directive and I am emotionally and mentally capable to make the health care decisions contained in this directive.

(f) I understand that before I sign this directive, I can add to or delete from or otherwise change the wording of this directive and that I may add to or delete from this directive at any time and that any changes shall be consistent with Washington state law or federal constitutional law to be legally valid.

(g) It is my wish that every part of this directive be fully implemented. If for any reason any part is held invalid it is my wish that the remainder of my directive be implemented.

(h) I make the following additional instructions regarding my care:

SIGN YOUR NAME AND PRINT YOUR ADDRESS

Signed: _____

City, County, and State of Residence: _____

_____

WITNESSING PROCEDURE

———

TWO WITNESSES SIGN HERE

The declarer has been personally known to me and I believe him or her to be capable of making health care decisions.

Witness: _____

Witness: _____

© 2000
PARTNERSHIP FOR
CARING, INC.

Courtesy of **Partnership for Caring, Inc.**   6/96
1620 Eye Street, NW, Suite 202, Washington, DC 20006 800-989-9455

INSTRUCTIONS

WASHINGTON
DURABLE POWER OF ATTORNEY FOR HEALTH CARE

I understand that my wishes as expressed in my living will may not cover all possible aspects of my care if I become incapacitated. Consequently, there may be a need for someone to accept or refuse medical intervention on my behalf, in consultation with my physician. Therefore,

PRINT YOUR NAME

I, _____, as principal, designate and appoint the person(s) listed below as my attorney-in-fact for health care decisions.

First Choice: Name: _____

Address: _____

City/State/Zip Code: _____

_____

Telephone Number: _____

PRINT THE NAME, ADDRESS AND TELEPHONE NUMBER OF YOUR FIRST CHOICE TO ACT AS YOUR ATTORNEY-IN-FACT

If the above person is unable, unavailable, or unwilling to serve, I designate:

Second Choice: Name: _____

Address: _____

City/State/Zip Code: _____

_____

Telephone Number: _____

PRINT THE NAME, ADDRESS AND TELEPHONE NUMBER OF YOUR SECOND CHOICE TO ACT AS YOUR ATTORNEY-IN-FACT

1.   This Power of Attorney shall take effect upon my incapacity to make my own health care decisions, as determined by my treating physician and one other physician, and shall continue as long as the incapacity lasts or until I revoke it, whichever happens first.

2.   The powers of my attorney-in-fact under this Power of Attorney are limited to making decisions about my health care on my behalf. These powers shall include the power to order the withholding or

| WASHINGTON DURABLE POWER OF ATTORNEY FOR HEALTH CARE — PAGE 2 OF 2 |

ADD PERSONAL INSTRUCTIONS (IF ANY)

withdrawal of life-sustaining treatment if my attorney-in-fact believes, in his or her own judgment, that is what I would want if I could make the decision myself. The existence of this Durable Power of Attorney for Health Care shall have no effect upon the validity of any other Power of Attorney for other purposes that I have executed or may execute in the future.

3.   In the event that a proceeding is initiated to appoint a guardian of my person under RCW 11.88, I nominate the person designated as my first choice (on page 1) to serve as my guardian. My second choice (on page 1) will serve as my guardian if the first person is unable or unwilling.

4.   I make the following additional instructions regarding my care:

By signing this document, I indicate that I understand the purpose and effect of this Durable Power of Attorney for Health Care.

SIGN AND DATE YOUR DOCUMENT

Dated this _____ day of _____, 20_____.
                      (date)   *(month)*   *(year)*

Signed: _____

WITNESSING PROCEDURE
———

TWO WITNESSES SIGN HERE

The person named as principal in this document is personally known to me. I believe that he/she is of sound mind, and that he/she signed this document freely and voluntarily.

Witness: _____

Witness: _____

© 2000
PARTNERSHIP FOR CARING, INC.

Courtesy of **Partnership for Caring, Inc.**   6/96
1620 Eye Street, NW, Suite 202, Washington, DC 20006 800-989-9455

The Living Bank Uniform Anatomical Gift Act Donor Form

For more information about organ/tissue donation, contact The Living Bank at 1-800-528-2971.

The organ and tissue shortage is a crisis, but it is a crisis with a cure. Remember, the only way your family will know your decision is if you tell them.

Donor Name _____

Address _____

City/State/Zip _____

In the hope that I might help others, I make this anatomical gift, if medically acceptable, to take effect upon my death. I give any needed organs and tissue.

Donor Signature _____

Social Security Number_____

Date _____

Witness #1 _____

Witness #2 _____

Next of Kin _____

Relationship to Donor _____

Next of Kin Address _____

Next of Kin City/State/Zip_____

Next of Kin Phone(s) _____

Next of Kin Signature _____

The Living Bank P.O. Box 6725 Houston, Texas 77265 1-800-528-2971

Mail this filled-out form to the address above. The Living Bank will send you complete information and your donor card to carry with you in the event of an emergency. Feel free to copy and use this form for family members.

_____ Check here if you do not want to receive quarterly informational newsletters from the Living Bank.

_____ Check here if you would like additional donor registration forms sent to you by The Living Bank. Include a voluntary contribution to cover the cost. Please specify quantity.

Currently, there is NO national nor state registry to list those individuals wishing to be organ donors. That is why it is VITAL that you inform your next of kin of your desire to donate. The following card may be printed, filled out, and retained for your records.

UNIFORM DONOR CARD

In the hope that I may help others, I hereby make this anatomical gift, if medically acceptable, to take effect upon my death. The following indicates my desires:

I give

(a)_____any needed organs or tissues

or

(b)_____only the following organs or tissues

_____
(Specify the organ(s) or tissue(s))

for the purposes of transplantation, therapy, medical research or education.

_____
Signature of Donor

_____
Signature of Witness

_____/_____/_____
Date Signed

_____
City and State

This is a legal document under the Uniform Anatomical Gift Act or other similar laws.

Please remember to inform your loved ones about your decision to donate.

California Transplant Donor Network
888-570-9400

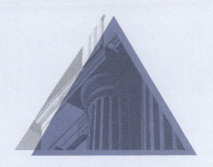

Bibliography

Allison, M: Forum Airs Issues in Human Genetics: Institute Sponsored Free Event. The Seattle Times, B1, May 22, 2005.

American College of Physicians-American Society of Internal Medicine: Educational Requirements for License Renewal (Continuing Medical Education) (2001) [Online]. Available: http://www.acponline.org/cme/licenses.html

American College of Physicians-American Society of Internal Medicine: Guidelines from Malpractice Insurers? (ACP-ASIM Observer) [Online]. Available: http://www.acponline.org/journals/new/nov98/insurers.html

American Medical Association: Allied Health and Rehabilitation Professions Education Directory, 2000–2001.

American Medical Association (AMA): Legal Issues: Professional Liability Insurance (2001) [Online]. Available: http://www.ama-assn.org/ama/pub/category/4583.html

American Academy of Pediatrics: Immunization Protects Children 2006 Immunization Schedule (2006)[Online]. Available: http://www.cispimmunize.org/

Angel, RJ: Cultural Sensitivity—Who needs it? The Gerontologist, 39(3):376–378, 1999.

Bailey, DM, and Schwartzberg, SL: Ethical and Legal Dilemmas in Occupational Therapy. FA Davis, Philadelphia, 1995.

Baron, CH: In Brief: Not DEA'd yet: Gonzales v. Oregon. Hastings Center Report 36(2): 8, 2006.

Bloodborne Pathogens and Needlestick Prevention: 2006. [Online] Available: http://www.osha.gov/SLTC/bloodbornepathogens/index.html

Borglum, KC, and Cate, DM: Medical Practice Forms: Every Form You Need to Succeed, ed 3. Practice Management Information Corp (PMIC), California, 2003.

Boyce, N, and Kaplan, DE: The God game no more: The feds crack down on a human cloning lab: U.S. News and World Report, 131(2):20–21, 2001.

Brant, M, and Evan, T: Reality Check for Roe. Newsweek, 44–45, March 6, 2006.

Bridges, A: Deaths renew call for ban on RU-486: The Kitsap Sun, Saturday, March 18, 2006; A4.

Brow, JA: When Culture and Medicine Collide. Professional Medical Assisting 34(1): 8–10, 2001.

Brown, K: The human genome business today. Scientific America 283(1):50–56, 2000.

Burton, BK: Quick Guide to HIPAA for the Physician's Office. Saunders: Elsevier Science (USA), Missouri, 2004.

Caplan, J: The new front line in abortion wars. Time 167(10):10, March 6, 2006.

Carey, B: Serious about security: Consumer groups laud new rules guarding privacy of medical records: The Seattle Times, Scene, May 6, 2001.

Cascardo, DC: Medical office manager: Resolve billing problems before they start. Professional Medical Assisting 34(4): Jul/Aug 2001.

Chang, CF, Price, SA, and Pfoutz, SK: Economics and Nursing: Critical Professional Issues. FA Davis, Philadelphia, 2001.

Chiong, W: Brain death without definitions. Hastings Center Report 35(6):20–30, 2005.

Chop, WC, and Robnett, RH: Gerontology for the Healthcare Professional. FA Davis, Philadelphia, 1999.

Church, GM: Genomes for all. Scientific American 294(1):47–54, January 2006.

Code of Medical Ethics: Current Opinions with annotations 2004-2005, American Medical Association, AMA Press, 2004.

Colburn, D: Other states see path in ruling on assisted suicide. The Sunday Oregonian, A-11, January 22, 2006.

Cole, W: Seed of controversy. Time 153(1):77, 1999.

Davidoff, F: Sex, politics, and morality at the FDA: Reflections on the Plan B decision. Hastings Center Report 35(32):20–25, March-April 2006.

Desmon, S: Tribal leader proposes abortion clinic: The Seattle Times, A-5, April 2, 2006.

DeVaro, E, and Turner, L: Research notes: Values in managed care. Hastings Center Report 27(1):48, 1997.

Diller, L: Fallout from the pharma scandals: The loss of doctors' credibility? Hastings Center Report 35(3):28–29, 2005.

Drench, ME, Noonan, AC, Sharby, N, and Ventura, SH: Psychosocial Aspects of Health Care. Practice Hall, New Jersey, 2003.

Dresser, R: Human cloning and the FDA. Hastings Center Report 33(3):7–8, May-June 2003.

Dresser, R: A new era in drug regulation? Hastings Center Report 35(3):10–11, May-June 2005.

Dresser, R: Schiavo's legacy: The need for an objective standard. Hastings Center Report 35(3):20–22, 2005.

Edge, RS, and Groves, JR: Ethics of Health Care: A Guide for Clinical Practice, ed 3. Thomson–Delmar Learning, New York, 2006.

Eitioni, A: Medical Records: Enhancing Privacy, Preserving the Common Good. Hastings Center Report 29(2):14–23, 1999.

Ellis, JR, and Hartley, CL: Nursing in Today's World: Trends, Issues, and Management ed 8. Lippincott Williams and Wilkins, New York, 2004.

Emanual, EJ: Justice and managed care: Four principles for the just allocation of health care. Hastings Center Report, 8–16, May–June 2000.

Ezzell, C: The business on the human genome. Scientific America 283(1):64, 2000.

Faden, R: The advisory committee on human radiation experiments: Reflections on a presidential commission. Hastings Center Report 26(5):5, 1996.

Fields, H: What comes next? Scientists are now grappling with a major setback to stem cell research. U.S. News and World Report, 56–58, January 23, 2006.

Fineman, H, and Evan, T: "The GOP's abortion anxiety." Newsweek, 24–29, March 20, 2006.

Fischman, J: Drug bazaar: Getting medicine off the web is easy, but dangerous. U.S. News and World Report 126(24): 1999.

Flight, M: Law, Liability, and Ethics for Medical Office Professionals, ed 4. Thompson–Delmar Learning, New York, 2004.

Fordyce, M: Geriatric Pearls. FA Davis, Philadelphia, 1999.

Fregman, BF: Medical Law and Ethics, ed 2. Pearson Prentice Hall, New Jersey, 2006.

Frisch, NC, and Frisch, LE: Psychiatric Mental Health Nursing, ed 3. Thomson–Delmar Learning, New York, 2006.

Furrow, BR, Greaney, TL, Johnson, SH, Jost, T, and Schwartz, RL: Health Law: Practitioner Treatise Series, 1 (Chapters 1–10). West Publishing Company, Minnesota, 1995.

Furrow, BR, Greaney, TL, Johnson, SH, Jost, TS, Schwartz, RL: Health Law, ed 2, Vol. 1. West Group, Minnesota, 2000.

Furrow, BR, Greaney, TL, Johnson, SH, Jost, TS, and Schwartz, RL: Health Law, ed 2, Vol. 2. West Group, Minnesota, 2000.

Furrow, BR, Greaney, TL, Johnson, SH, Jost, TS, and Schwartz, RL: Bioethics: Health Care Law and Ethics, ed 5. Thomson, Minnesota, 2001.

Gabard, DL, and Martin, MW: Physical Therapy Ethics. FA Davis Company, Philadelphia, 2003.

Gilgoff, D: A break in the ranks. U S News and World Report 140(9):32, March 13, 2006.

Golden, F: Good eggs, bad eggs. Time 153(1):56–59, 1999.

Gorman, C: Drugs by design. Time 153(1):78–83, 1999.

Graves, B, and Colburn, D: Why this pill costs you $7.14. The Sunday Oregonian, A-1, April 30, 2006.

Guido, GW: Legal and Ethical Issues in Nursing, ed 3. Prentice Hall, New Jersey, 2001.

Harris, DM: Contemporary Issues in Healthcare Law and Ethics, ed 2. Aupha-HAP, Washington, DC, 2003.

Healy, M: Close up: Bartering for their lives… The Seattle Times, A-3, Sunday, November 7, 2004.

Heath, D, and Wilson, D: Uninformed consent: What patients at "The Hutch" weren't told about the experiments in which they did, Part 1 and 2. The Seattle Times, March 11, 2001.

Hoffmaster, B: What does vulnerability mean? Hastings Center Report 36(2):38–45, 2006.

Human Genome to go public. CNN [Online], February 9, 2001. Available: http://www.cnn.com/2001/HEALTH/02/09/genome.results/

Jaroff, L: Fixing the genes: Time 153(1):68–73, 1999.

Jones, HW, and Cohen J: State of general purpose. Fertility and Sterility 81(5), Suppl. 4, May 2004.

Jonsen, AR: Bioethics Beyond the Headlines: Who Lives? Who Dies? Who Decides? Rowman and Littlefield Publishers, Inc, New York, 2005.

Judson, K, and Hicks, S: Glencoe Law and Ethics for Medical Careers, ed 3. Glencoe McGraw-Hill, New York, 2003.

Kaebnick, GE (Ed.): The next set of questions about stem cells. The Hastings Center Report 36(1): January-February 2006.

Kaplan, S, and Brownlee, S: Dying for a Cure: Why Cancer patients often turn to risky, experimental treatments-and wind up paying with their lives. U.S. News and World Report 127(14): 1999.

Kelleher, S, and Wilson, D: Suddenly sick: The hidden big business behind your doctor's diagnosis. The Seattle Times: Post Intelligencer, A-1, June 26, 2005.

Klab, C: DNA and the Secrets of Who We Are. Newsweek, 46–55, February 6, 2006.

Kline, RM: Biotech: Stem cell research. Scientific American 284(4): April, 2001.

Kluger, J: Who owns our genes. Time 153(1):51, 1999.

Lalli, W: Avoid replacement pains: Nurture the staff you have. CMA Today, May-Jun, 2006.

Lanza, R, and Rosenthal, N: The stem cell challenge. Scientific American 290(6):93–99, June 2004.

Lauritzen, P, McClure, M, Smith, ML, and Trew, A: The gift of life and the common good: The need for a communal approach to organ procurement. Hastings Center Report 31(1):29–35, 2001.

Lemonick, MD: Designer Babies. Time 153(1):64–66, 1999.

Lemonick, MD: On the horizon: Tomorrow's tissue factory. Time 153(1):89–90, 1999.

Lemonick, MD, and Thompson, D: Racing to map our DNA. Time 153(1):44–50, 1999.

Lemonick, MD: The rise and fall of the cloning king. Time 167(2): January 9, 2006.

Lindh, WQ, Pooler, MS, Tamparo, CD, and Cerrato, JU: Comprehensive Medical Assisting: Administrative and Clinical Competencies. Delmar Publishers, New York, 1998.

Lindh, WQ, Pooler, MS, Tamparo, CD, and Dahl, BM: Administrative Medical Assisting, ed 3. Thomson–Delmar Learning, New York, 2006.

Locate A Bank: Sperm Banking Directory.com: A National Directory of Sperm Cryobanks, 2001. Available: http://www.spermbankdirectory.com

Mahdoubi, KF: Schiavo's legacy: Health directives registry proposed. The Kitsap Sun, 2, February 15, 2006.

Marcus, DL: Mothers with another's eggs: As demand for donors accelerates, questions on the price of a child. Science and Ideas, April 12, 1999.

Mathis, RL, and Jackson, JH: Human Resource Management, ed 9. South-Western College Publishing, Cincinnati, Ohio, 2000.

McCabe, ERB: Medical genetics. JAMA 275(23):1, 1996.

McCormack, J: Exit interviews: Proceed with caution and courtesy. CMA Today, Sep-Oct 2004.

Medical Ethical Advisor: Should you or shouldn't you? What to do when parents ask you to keep secrets: MEA 17(4):37–48, 2001.

Medical Group Management Association (2006) [Online]. Available: http://www.mgma.com/

Medical Office Manager: HIPAA's final regulations: Access your readiness. PMA, AAMA, 32(4):24–25, Jun/Aug 1999.

Mooney, DJ, and Mikos, AG: Growing new organs. Scientific America 280(4):65, 1999.

Morrison, M: Who's leading the way? Parade, 4–5, July 10, 2005.

Mozam, F: Families, patients, and physicians in medical decisionmaking: A Pakistani perspective: Hastings Center Report, 28–37, November–December 2000.

NARAL:Pro-Choice America. Fetal Tissue Research: Moving Beyond Anti-Choice Politics.

[Online] January 1, 2004. Available: www.naral.org/facts/fetal_tissue_research.cfm? renderforprint=1

Neergaard, L: Korean scientist announce major stem cell progress: The new cells genetically match sick patients. The Kitsap Sun, C-1, June 20, 2005.

Occupational Outlook Handbook, 2004–2005 Edition, U.S. Department of Labor, Bureau of Statistics, Bulletin 2570, Superintendent of Documents, U.S. Government Printing Office, Washington, DC, 2004.

O'Keefe, ME: Nursing Practice and the Law: Avoiding Malpractice and other Legal Risks. FA Davis, Philadelphia, 2001.

Ostling, RN: Ethics of stem-cell research present thorny dilemma for religious leaders. The Kitsap Sun, A-5, June 5, 2005.

Our Bodies, Ourselves: A New Edition for a New Era—The Boston Women's Health Book Collective. A Touchstone Book, New York, 2005.

Pedersen, RA: Stem cells for medicine. Scientific America, 280(4):69–73, 1999.

Pozgar, GD: Legal Aspects of Health Care Administration. Jones and Bartlett Publishers, Massachusetts, 2004.

Pozgar, GD: Legal and Ethical Issues for Health Professionals. Jones and Bartlett Publishers, Massachusetts, 2005.

Purnell, LD, and Paulanka, BJ: Transcultural Health Care: A Culturally Competent Approach. FA Davis, Philadelphia, 1998.

Quinn, JB: The health-care lottery's winners and losers. Newsweek, 47, February 27, 2006.

Rojas-Burke, J: Comparison shopping moves to medicine. The Sunday Oregonian, E-4, January 22, 2006.

Saletan, W: Life after Roe. The Seattle Times, D-5, April 30, 2006; Opinion, Local.

Schiff, L: Supreme Court: Government can't bar late-term abortions: Medical Economics 63(8):16, 2000.

Schonwald, J: A guide to genetic testing and counseling. Professional Medical Assisting, 17–21, November/December 2001.

Schrof, JM: Miracle vaccines: Advances in genetic engineering are spawning a new generation of powerful disease fighters. U.S. News and World Report 125(20): 1998.

Sierpina, VS: Integrative Health Care: Complementary and Alternative Therapies for the Whole Person. FA Davis, Philadelphia, 2001.

Siminoff, LA, and Chillag, K: The fallacy of the "gift of life." Hastings Center Report 29(6):34–41, 1999.

Spielberg, AR: Online without a net: Physician-patient communication by electronic mail: American Journal of Law and Medicine, 25(2/3):267–295, 1999.

Spielberg, AR: On call and online: Sociohistorical, legal, and ethical implications of E-mail for the patient-physician relationship: JAMA, 280(15):1353–1359, 1998.

Stein, Rob: Search for transplant organs becomes web free-for-all, The Kitsap Sun.

Stix, G: Owning the stuff of life. Scientific American 294(1):76–83, February 2006.

Stolberg, SG: Politicians grapple with stem-cell issue: The Seattle Times, News, Sunday July 1, 2001.

Streisand, B: Who's your daddy? U.S. News and World Report, 53–56, February 13, 2006.

Sutcliffe, AJ: Current Issues in the Diagnosis of Brain Stem Death. Presented at the 17th Annual Trauma Anesthesia and Critical Care Symposium, Sydney, Australia, October 15–17, 2004.

Szegedy-Maszek, M: A lesson before dying: Med schools tackle end-of-life issues. U.S. World News and World Report, 48–49, 2001.

Taber's Cyclopedic Medical Dictionary (19th Ed.): FA Davis, Philadelphia, 2001.

Tesch, DJ, Dunnington, N, and Howard, CH: Washington Medical Records for the 21st Century: Medical Educational Services Inc., Eau Claire, Wisconsin, 2001.

The Editors: The promise of tissue engineering: Special report: Scientific America 280(4):59, 1999.

The White House: President Signs "Stem Cell Therapeutic and Research Act of 2005." [Online] December 20, 2005. Available: www.whitehouse.gov/news/releases/2005/12/20051220-1.html

Thomas, D: Positioning Your Practice for the Managed Care Market. Williams & Wilkins, Baltimore, 1996.

Thompson, D: Gene maverick: Time 153(1):54–55, 1999.

Timmerman, L, and Heath, D: Drug researchers leak secrets to Wall St. The Seattle Times: Sunday Post-Intelligencer, A-1, August 7, 2006.

Tong, R: New Perspectives in Healthcare Ethics: An Interdisciplinary and Crosscultural Approach. Pearson–Prentice Hill, New Jersey, 2007.

Tumulty, K: Where the real action is. Time 167(5):50–51, January 30, 2006.

U.S. Department of Justice: Americans with Disabilities Act (ADA): Enforcing the ADA-Update, January–March 2001.

Verrengia, JB: Ethicists bark about cloned dog. The Kitsap Sun, A-2, August, 4, 2005.

Washington Physician's Guide to Health Law. Washington Medical Association, ed 2. Washington State Medical Association, Washington, 2001.

Washington State Vital Statistics 1999: Washington State Department of Health Center for Health Statistics, April 2001.

Washington Weekly. The Rutherford Institute, Jan. 16, 1997. National Bioethics Advisory Commission meets in Washington, D.C.

Weiss, R: The power to divide. National Geographic Magazine, 3–27, July 2005.

Wilson, BG: Ethics and Basic Law: For Medical Imaging Professionals. FA Davis, Philadelphia, 1997.

Woodward, C: Gov. Gregoire enacts statewide registry for end-of-life wishes. The Kitsap Sun, A-8, March 18, 2006.

Wolfson, J: Erring on the side of Theresa Schiavo: Reflections of the special guardian ad litem. Hastings Center Report 35(3):16–19, 2006.

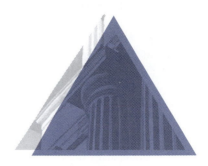

Index

A